ALSO BY STAN MACK

The Story of the Jews: A 4,000-Year Adventure

Stan Mack's Real Life American Revolution

Heartbreak and Roses (with Janet Bode)

Hard Time (with Janet Bode)

For Better, For Worse (with Janet Bode)

10 Bears in My Bed

Janet & Me

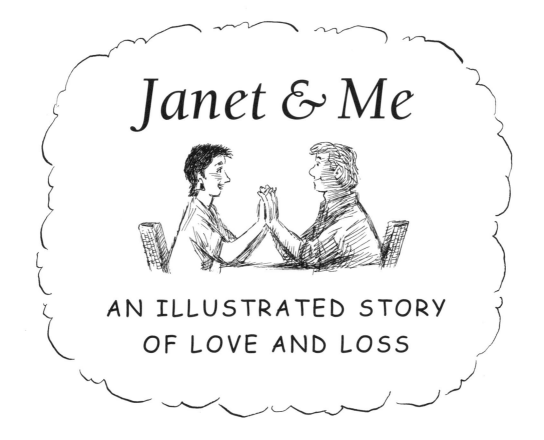

AN ILLUSTRATED STORY
OF LOVE AND LOSS

STAN MACK

SIMON & SCHUSTER PAPERBACKS
New York   London   Toronto   Sydney

SIMON & SCHUSTER PAPERBACKS
Rockefeller Center
1230 Avenue of the Americas
New York, NY 10020

First Simon & Schuster paperback edition 2004

SIMON & SCHUSTER PAPERBACKS and colophon are registered trademarks
of Simon & Schuster, Inc.

"Look Up, Look Down That Lonesome Road": Traditional,
arranged and adapted by Gaither Carlton, as sung by
Doc Watson, copyright © Hillgreen Music.

"Save Your Tears": copyright © 1977, Carole Mayedo.

For information about special discounts for bulk purchases,
please contact Simon & Schuster Special Sales:
1-800-456-6798 or business@simonandschuster.com

Designed by Helene Berinsky

Manufactured in the United States of America

1 3 5 7 9 10 8 6 4 2

Library of Congress Cataloging-in-Publication Data
Mack, Stanley.
Janet & me : an illustrated story of love and loss / Stan Mack—1st Simon & Schuster trade pbk. ed.
p. cm.
1. Bode, Janet—Health. 2. Breast—Cancer—Patients—New York (State)—New York—Biography. 3. Cancer—
Caricatures and cartoons. I. Title: Janet and me. II. Title.

RC280.B8B596 2004
362.96'99449"0092—dc22
[B]   2004052170
ISBN 0-684-87278-1 (pbk)

For Janet, of course

I never thought when we first met,
this awful day would come, my love…
The best of friends must part someday,
and why not you and I, my love.

"Look Up, Look Down That Lonesome Road"

Author's note

This is a true story. The people, their words, and the events described are real.

For brevity, except for Janet and me, I have identified people by their first names only. I have also changed the names of the health-care professionals who treated Janet and the name of the hospital where she was a patient. I have not changed the names of the hospice organization and its personnel who cared for her.

The readers will note that I have used the device of having some people speak directly to them from the margins of the pages. I interviewed these people after Janet's death. Their recollections are sifted through the filter of time.

I have attempted to present everyone's words and views as accurately as possible.

Regarding the many illustrations: drawing is my most personal language. I felt I could best bring the reader into Janet's and my world through pictures. Some drawings are more cartoony, others more realistic; as long as I felt the reader could recognize the characters, I let my hand and emotions find the right style. And, in the process, I discovered that sketching our neighborhood and apartment, portraying Janet and myself together during the good times and bad, depicting us talking to each other, helped me put painful memories to rest.

Acknowledgments

My deep thanks to my editors—to Melissa Possick, who first said, "Let's do it!" and then never wavered in her commitment, and to Sydny Miner, who took over at a critical time and guided me and this book with a sure and understanding hand. And to my agent, Gary Morris, who was always there to put things in perspective.

When I began work on this book, I decided to listen for Janet's voice in the memories of her friends and colleagues. And each one patiently sat with me and offered his or her recollections. They are listed alphabetically because, whether they contributed a great deal or only a small piece, every one immeasurably enriched this story. Also included in this list are health-care professionals to whom I turned to discuss medical issues Janet and I faced, and I appreciate the time they gave me. (However, this is a personal memoir and, while there is much to be learned, it is not intended as a source of medical expertise.)

Barbara Althoff, Joanne Althoff, Deborah Axelrod, Kristy Bakker, Bill Baum, Agnes Beck, Gloria Benjamin, Karl Bissinger, Sonya Blanco, Marlene Bloom, Molly Bloom, Paul Brenner, Rob and Lisa Brill, Jean Brown, Florrie Burke, Wendy Caplin, Chas Carner, Lucy Cefalu, Val and Ron Chernow, David Chesnick, Norris Chumley, Judy Daniels, Mariella Dearman, Karen deVries, Jeanne Dougherty and Bill Wood, Karen Dublin, Susan Dunn, Molly Eagan, Richard Eagan and Liz Ostrow, Kathy Ebel, Cliff Fagan, Marion Fay, Brian Fisher, Stewart Fleishman, Donna Forsman, Kay Franey, Jim Freydberg, Bridget Funk, Ellen Gold, Jane Goldberg, Meryl Gordon, Pat Gordon, Harriet and the late Ted Gottfried, Peggy Greene, Freeda Greer, Beverly Horowitz, Joan Athanas Kaufman, Joe Kelly, Kay Kelly,

Max Kelly, Kathryn Kilgore, Harriet King, Paul Krassner, Keith Kurman, Sally Lahm, Kathy Lawrence, Austin Long-Scott, Kenneth Mack and Stephanie Ripple, Peter Mack, Howard and Agnes Mauthe, Carole Mayedo, Rosemarie and Marvin Mazor, Pam McFarlane, Joy McKay, Betty Medsger and John Racanelli, Daniel Meltzer, Rick Meyerowitz, Joe Mohbat, Auda Moncion, Arlene Morales, Jane O'Reilly, Andrea Osnow, Sandra Payne, Daniel Pelavin, Judy Pollock, Russell Primm, Virginia Reath, Howie Rosen, Jill Rosenberg, Ellen Rubin, Connie Schlee, Ellen Schrecker and Marv Gettleman, David Seres, Mike Sexton, Peggy Sexton, Kathy Squires, the late Mary Jane Tacchi, San San Tin, Nell Ward and Sue Hardesty, and Marilou Blanco Yarosh.

As Janet's illness worsened and I was in danger of collapsing under the strain, there were four women to whom I could always turn for strength. They are Jane Ashe, Carolyn Bode, Linda Broessel, and Kate Sullivan. I will always love them for that.

And to my dear Susan Champlin, without whom, quite simply, I could not have written this book.

Contents

A String Without a Kite

This is the story of a love affair.

For eighteen years Janet Bode and I lived, worked, and traveled together. We were almost never apart. And we never married. She'd say, "Why fix it if it ain't broke?" And I enjoyed that little thrill of the illicit.

I wonder now whether, even if we had chosen marriage, I would have thought any more deeply about the implications of the marriage vows "In sickness and in health, till death do us part." Who thinks about sickness and death when you're starting a life together?

Janet was fun and exciting, and we were healthy and in love and that was plenty. We focused on our work—she as a writer of nonfiction books for teenagers, I as a cartoonist. The future would take care of itself.

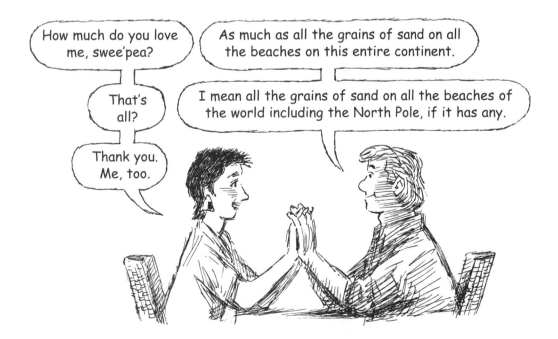

In those early days, I could never have imagined how much our relationship would transform my thinking about what was important in life, and what love is.

Little by little, as the years went by, and without at first realizing it, Janet and I built bridges to each other that would sustain us during the coming tough times.

In 1994, Janet was diagnosed with breast cancer.

Through the time of her illness, I learned to be both tender and strong. And when, as her condition worsened, I weakened, I also found I could recover. I now believe that a loving partner can help you find strengths within yourself that you didn't know were there.

When things got really bad, Janet continued to give me the trust that allowed me to help her; she even, I felt, showed me the way. Though I'd never taken care of a sick person and never heard the term "primary caregiver," that's what I did and that's what I became.

Janet stood up to her cancer and continued to embrace life. She fiercely held on to her belief in her own value—she refused to fade into neutral. She lost her temper, gossiped with friends, and made (sometimes bad) jokes about her disease. She never succumbed to despair. And she never stopped loving me.

Now I understand that the end is always part of the beginning. For every one of us, there will come a time of parting . . . and an afterwards. The love and values Janet and I built together were greater than the disease and would remain with me after her death. They are eternal. Janet lived for her season. Then, like a runner in a relay race, she passed on her love of life to me.

On December 30, 1999, about 6:30 a.m., one day before the end of the millennium, she died. Thankfully, it was in our home, our little loft in Greenwich Village, New York City. She was fifty-six years old.

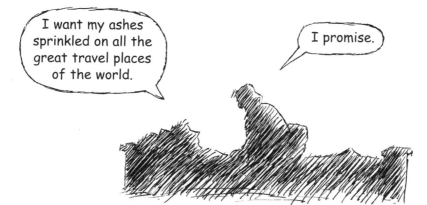

And then she was gone and there was no longer hope and no longer denial.

The following February, we held a memorial. Three hundred friends packed the cafeteria of our local grade school. Carole, a musician and friend of thirty years, sang a song about the time in 1970 when they'd left their husbands and hit the road in Mexico. Jane, the hoofer, tap-danced a eulogy. Howie, a trucker, revealed that Janet would sometimes drive his eighteen-wheeler on his interstate runs. And Phyllis, a librarian, spoke eloquently of how much teenagers loved Janet and her books.

I, too, spoke.

"I used to tell Janet she was like a brightly colored kite, flying high—but maybe a bit out of control. My job was to hold her string. Now the kite has gotten away from me. Not to crash, but to fly higher than I can see."

ME

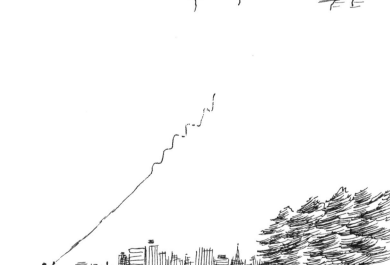

3

Eventually the memorial came to an end; and our friends said their good-byes.

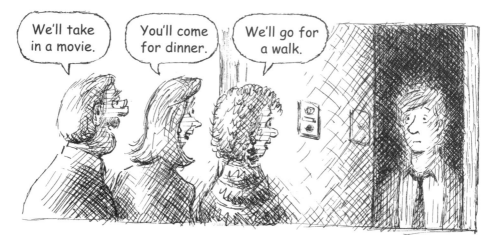

We'll take in a movie.

You'll come for dinner.

We'll go for a walk.

And I faced the heavy silence of our apartment. I couldn't bear sleeping in our bed, so I camped out on the floor. It was a familiar feeling.

We'd loved to travel, usually with a backpack apiece and a budget travel guidebook in hand. I thought about how, on our many trips abroad, she'd insisted on sleeping with me on floors—wood, tile, cement, didn't matter—rather than on the swaybacked mattresses we often found. I did it because of my bad back. She did it so I wouldn't be alone.

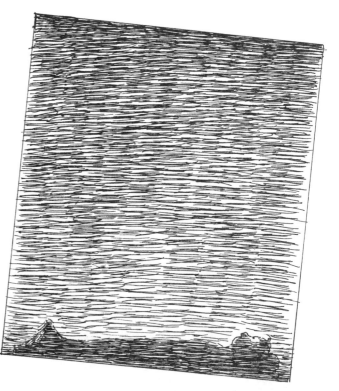

As the spring days went by, I stared out our window at the view Janet loved—the old Greenwich Village rooftops and, in the background twenty-four blocks north, the Empire State Building. Or I'd walk the neighborhood streets, imagining her coming toward me with that leggy, loose-limbed walk.

I remembered how we'd spot each other a half block away, and she'd smile with her big dark eyes. We'd come together and always manage to bump.

She reminded me of Olive Oyl in the Popeye comic strip. Shortly after we met, I began drawing her in my own cartoon strips. She loved it. I reprinted some of my drawings of her in the memorial brochure.

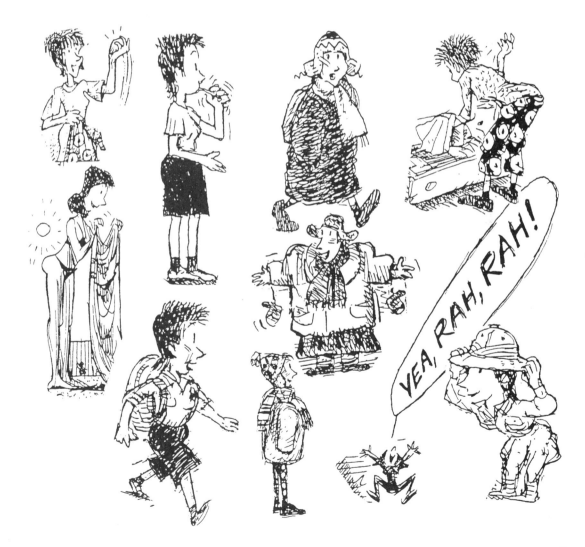

During those early months of grief, the monkey of death sat heavy on my shoulder.

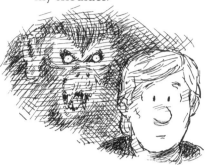

I measured my apartment building, wondering whether a six-story jump would be enough to kill me.

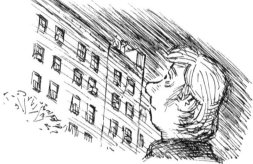

I was convinced my body held a cancer of its own.

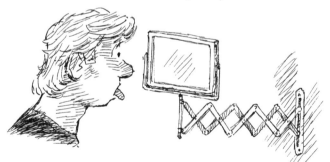

Bad memories kept crowding in, like the time I was sponging Janet and she looked down at her gaunt frame and said:

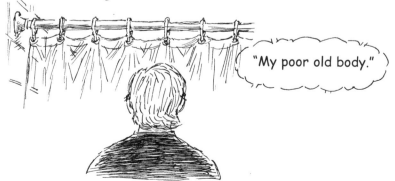

"My poor old body."

I thought about what the hospice brochure had said: "To dispel the fear of death is to make room for it in life." I intended someday to look squarely at her life and death. I would even welcome the pain. But not yet.

Meanwhile, I talked to Janet all the time. I knew exactly where she was.

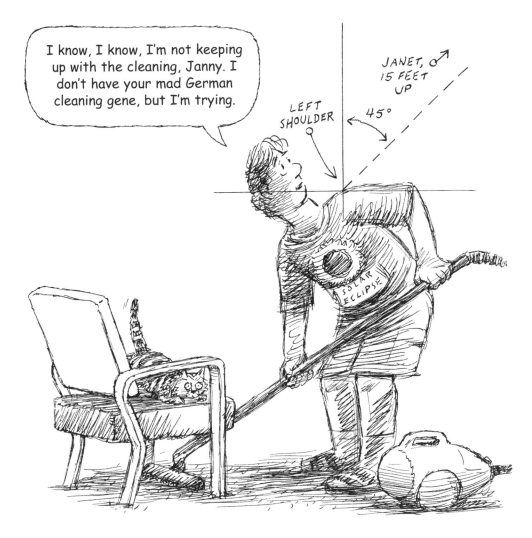

In August, as Janet and I had done every summer, I took the ferry to Fire Island to visit our friends Marvin and Rosemarie. On the ferry, the couple behind me was bickering. "Jerks!" I muttered.

At 6 p.m., I sat on the empty beach. There were the long blue shadows and the silvery light she knew I loved. From I don't know where, a big black dog lumbered up, settled down against my leg, and watched the waves with me. He was unexpectedly comforting. In time he wandered off, limping from an injured front paw.

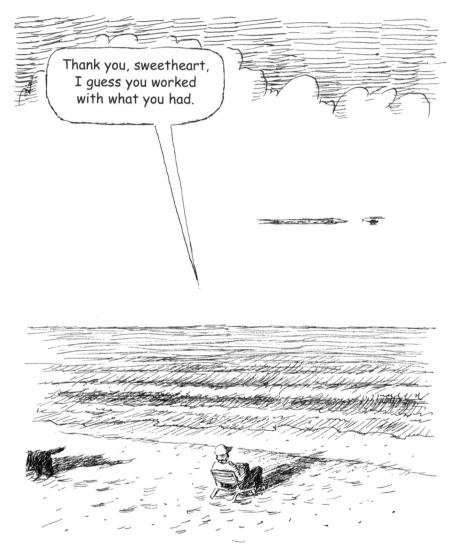

Thank you, sweetheart, I guess you worked with what you had.

By September, nine months after her death, the acute pain was receding, but I didn't want to forget anything about her.

It bothered me that I couldn't recall our everyday conversations. If we'd had such a great relationship, why couldn't I better remember? I wished I had a tape of our words that I could play back.

I did hear the words she'd said to me a few weeks before she died. They made me cry.

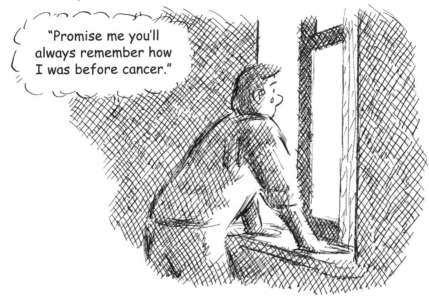

"Promise me you'll always remember how I was before cancer."

I thought about what made her special—her courage, her sense of outrage, her advocacy for teenagers, her quirkiness . . . and I could almost hear her saying, "You might mention that I was cute and a lot of fun, too."

I remembered her response early on when I began to include her in my comic strip, with me as the square-nosed guy with a mustache. She said, "I always knew I'd be famous, I just didn't know it would be in the funnies."

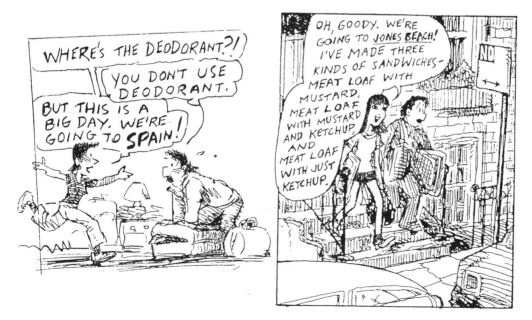

WHERE'S THE DEODORANT?!

YOU DON'T USE DEODORANT.

BUT THIS IS A BIG DAY. WE'RE GOING TO SPAIN!

OH, GOODY. WE'RE GOING TO JONES BEACH! I'VE MADE THREE KINDS OF SANDWICHES— MEAT LOAF WITH MUSTARD, MEAT LOAF WITH MUSTARD AND KETCHUP, AND MEAT LOAF WITH JUST KETCHUP.

This woman, whom I'd come to admire as well as love, had faced her illness the way she'd lived her life, with guts and charm. I was beginning to understand how I could keep her with me a while longer.

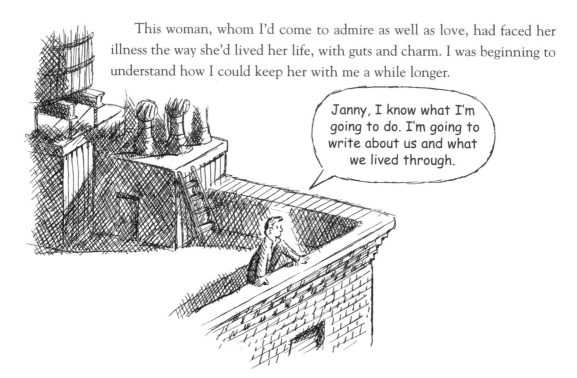

Janny, I know what I'm going to do. I'm going to write about us and what we lived through.

As Janet's disease progressed, she and I had talked about taking notes. We couldn't do it—which was ironic, since we'd always used "real life" in our work.

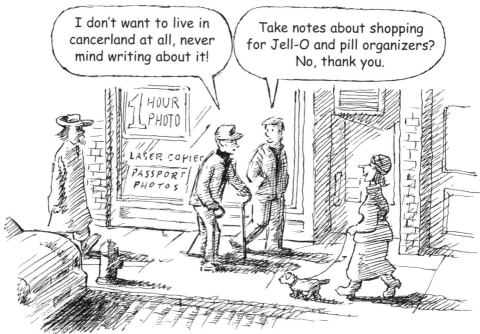

I don't want to live in cancerland at all, never mind writing about it!

Take notes about shopping for Jell-O and pill organizers? No, thank you.

But now I would search for her in her writings. I would discover her in the memories of her friends—especially among the ones I call the warrior women; those strong females who'd rallied around us when she was sick. And I would listen for her voice in my head.

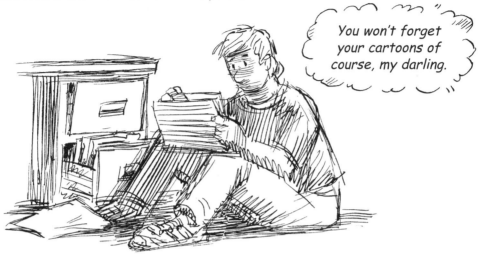

You won't forget your cartoons of course, my darling.

A book would also be a way to explore the everyday, unexpected, painful details that plagued us as her disease took hold and then worsened—and the human problems that the doctors would have us believe stopped short of their doors.

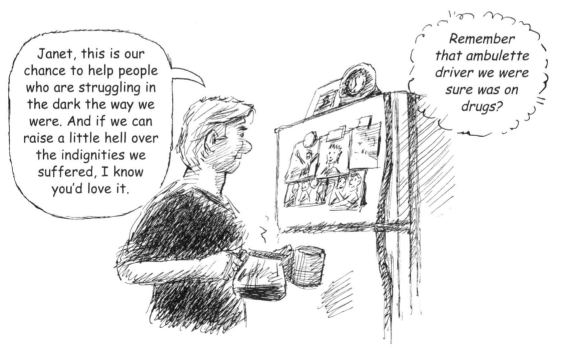

Janet, this is our chance to help people who are struggling in the dark the way we were. And if we can raise a little hell over the indignities we suffered, I know you'd love it.

Remember that ambulette driver we were sure was on drugs?

Janet's sister Carolyn worried that the project would be too painful for me.

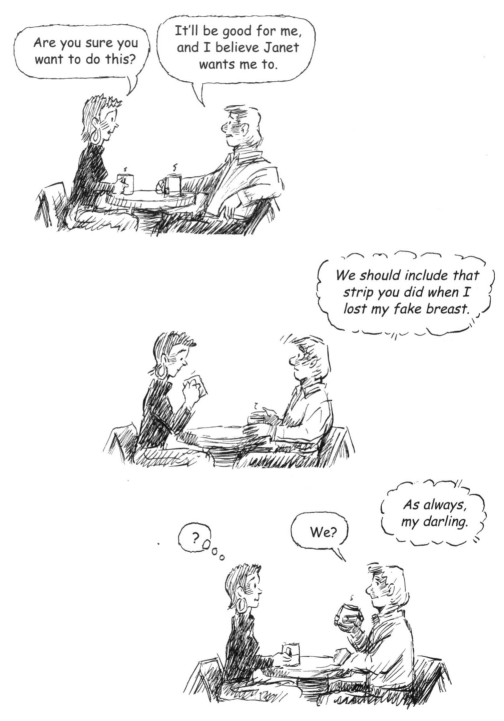

CHAPTER 1

Just a Zit

Whn Janet first felt the lump in her breast, she didn't tell me and didn't do anything about it for two months. She wasn't especially worried because her yearly mammograms had always been normal. And we were so busy, me with my strips, she finishing her new book for teens, *Death Is Hard to Live With*.

It wasn't until a letter arrived from a young reader, thanking Janet for her book on teen pregnancy, that she decided to act.

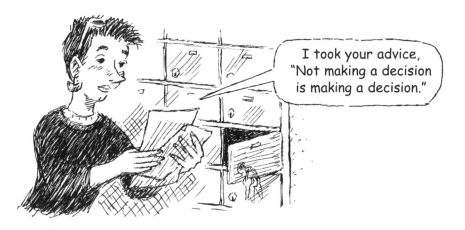

I took your advice, "Not making a decision is making a decision."

Janet didn't have a regular doctor because she'd always been healthy. For any checkups, she went to her friend Virginia, a physician's assistant. But Virginia was in the midst of moving and so she recommended an MD who examined Janet and sent her for a mammogram.

The letter from the breast diagnostic institute, which provided the results, said they'd found some irregularity. Included with their report was a list of recommended surgeons. Janet chose one who was on her insurance plan and went in for a biopsy.

I remember clearly that it was a bright, sunny day when we made our way to the hospital for the results. Janet talked about the two other women from her writers' group who had already been diagnosed with cancer.

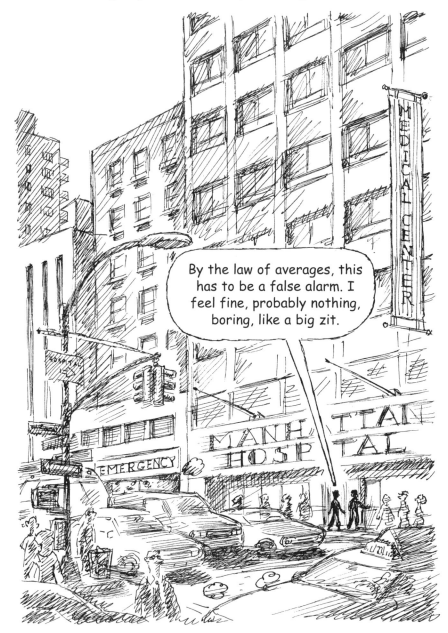

By the law of averages, this has to be a false alarm. I feel fine, probably nothing, boring, like a big zit.

The surgeon met us in a busy and narrow corridor just off the main lobby. There, opposite the cashier's office, he gave us the bad news . . . and rushed off. His abruptness was so unnerving we could hardly absorb the diagnosis.

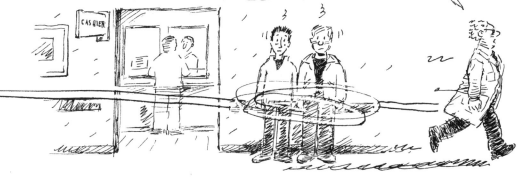

> Unfortunately, there's nowhere else to talk, and there's no nice way to say this. It's cancer. If you make an appointment with my secretary, we can talk about surgery.

We left the hospital looking for a lighthearted way to talk about information that was too new, too scary, too shocking to face directly.

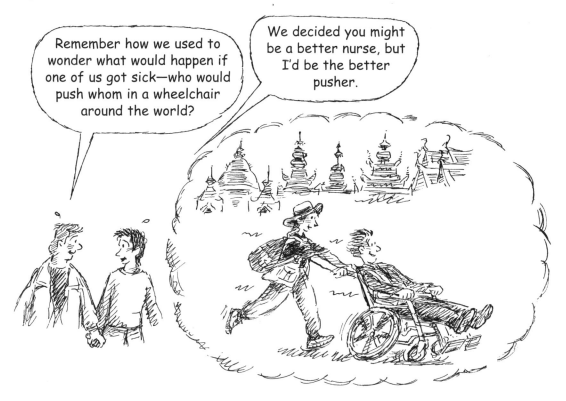

> Remember how we used to wonder what would happen if one of us got sick—who would push whom in a wheelchair around the world?

> We decided you might be a better nurse, but I'd be the better pusher.

Janet didn't seem to have a self-pity gene. First she minimized the cancer. She wrote in her diary that week, "I am bummed out!" Then she got angry at the universe and moved into a practical high gear. She spread her net wide, looking up organizations, experts, and publications, familiarizing herself with the disease.

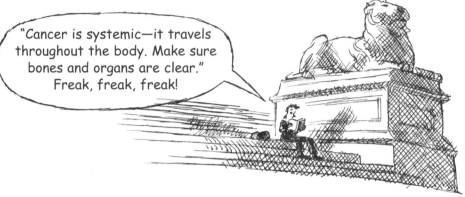

"Cancer is systemic—it travels throughout the body. Make sure bones and organs are clear."
Freak, freak, freak!

She also called friends who tried different ways of cheering her up.

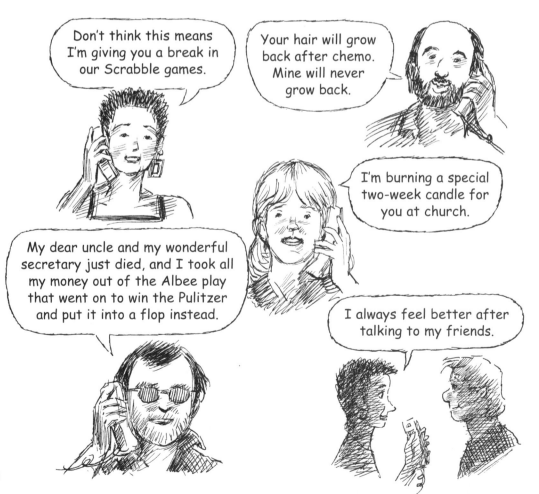

Don't think this means I'm giving you a break in our Scrabble games.

Your hair will grow back after chemo. Mine will never grow back.

I'm burning a special two-week candle for you at church.

My dear uncle and my wonderful secretary just died, and I took all my money out of the Albee play that went on to win the Pulitzer and put it into a flop instead.

I always feel better after talking to my friends.

A few days later we met with the surgeon, who recommended a mastectomy. He said he knew Janet would grieve for her breast and be anxious for reconstruction. Janet and I resented his paternalism and his assumptions. We left determined to find a different surgeon, one she could relate to.

Janet again called her friend Virginia.

"I met Janet at a women's health conference in '85. I loved her sexy *joie de vivre* and we became buddies. We used to compare notes on boyfriends and the question of having children.

"She said to me, 'Remember, kid, you can't go by conventional guidelines. You and I live on the fringes.'

"Janet had the body arrogance of the very healthy. Illness happened to other people. When she called, her tone was flip. But I knew her well enough to know that the diagnosis had been a real kick in the head."

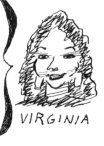

VIRGINIA

Virginia, I have breast cancer. So *au courant*. Also a nuisance.

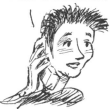

She'll work it out. I'm calling her.

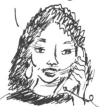

She's not his patient. And she's an amazing woman.

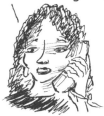

Janet, you're going to my friend Beverly. She's an excellent breast surgeon and you'll like each other.

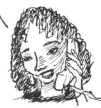

Beverly, you have to see this woman as a patient.

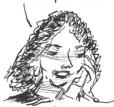

I'm very busy.

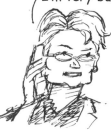

I like that she's a woman, but she's not on my insurance plan.

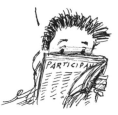

I don't have time, and she's another surgeon's patient.

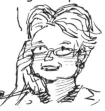

Just shut up and meet her!

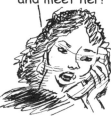

"Janet was charming, positive, and obviously comfortable with me. Some women are overwhelmed by their cancer. She was herself overwhelming. I was won over.

"We had a breast cancer chat. Her tumor was large-ish, she was small-breasted, and the margins around the tumor had tested positive, so we decided on mastectomy.

"We also discussed cosmetic surgery, which Janet rejected.

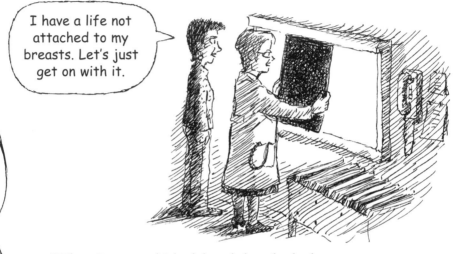

I have a life not attached to my breasts. Let's just get on with it.

BEVERLY

"When I operated I had found that she had an aggressive cancer with five lymph nodes involved, though I thought it was at an early stage and treatable. After the mastectomy, Janet was her usual unflappable self."

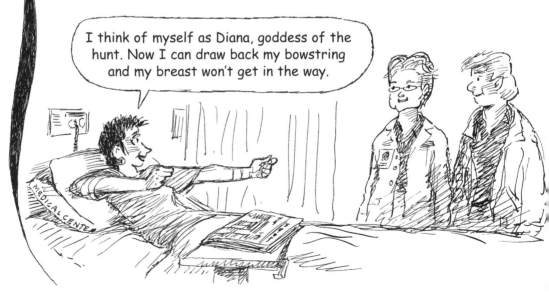

I think of myself as Diana, goddess of the hunt. Now I can draw back my bowstring and my breast won't get in the way.

Beverly recommended an oncologist, Laura. Janet and Laura met and immediately hit it off. Laura appreciated Janet's candor, but her own words seemed studied and nonspecific, always leaving us with handholds on hope.

"Janet's directness hit me in the face. She wanted straight talk, not euphemisms. I told her there was no way to predict the outcome, but that cancer can be controlled."

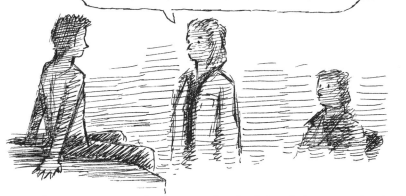

Janet, you have a high risk of future recurrence, but chemo, radiation, and hormonal therapies can significantly reduce that risk . . . everyone's biology is different—lots of women in your category are doing well.

LAURA

Laura set up an eleven-month schedule of chemo and radiation. Janet, reporter's notebook in hand, would press Laura for details about everything from side effects to insurance issues. But there was one question we never seemed to hear the answer to. Was it truly impossible to know? Was Laura's response ambiguous? Or did we just refuse to consider the idea of death?

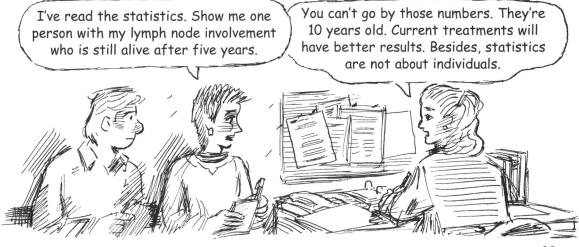

I've read the statistics. Show me one person with my lymph node involvement who is still alive after five years.

You can't go by those numbers. They're 10 years old. Current treatments will have better results. Besides, statistics are not about individuals.

Whatever the truth, Janet went into cancer treatment having decided she was going to live.

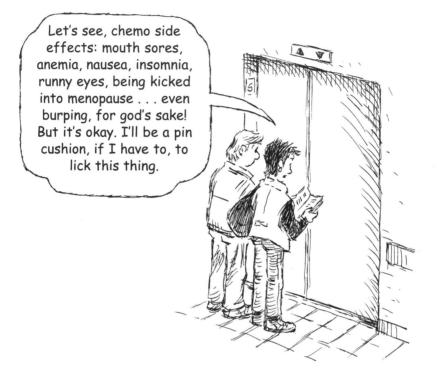

Let's see, chemo side effects: mouth sores, anemia, nausea, insomnia, runny eyes, being kicked into menopause . . . even burping, for god's sake! But it's okay. I'll be a pin cushion, if I have to, to lick this thing.

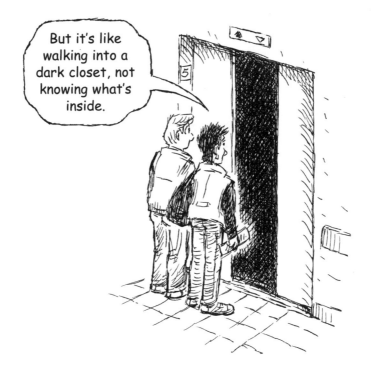

21

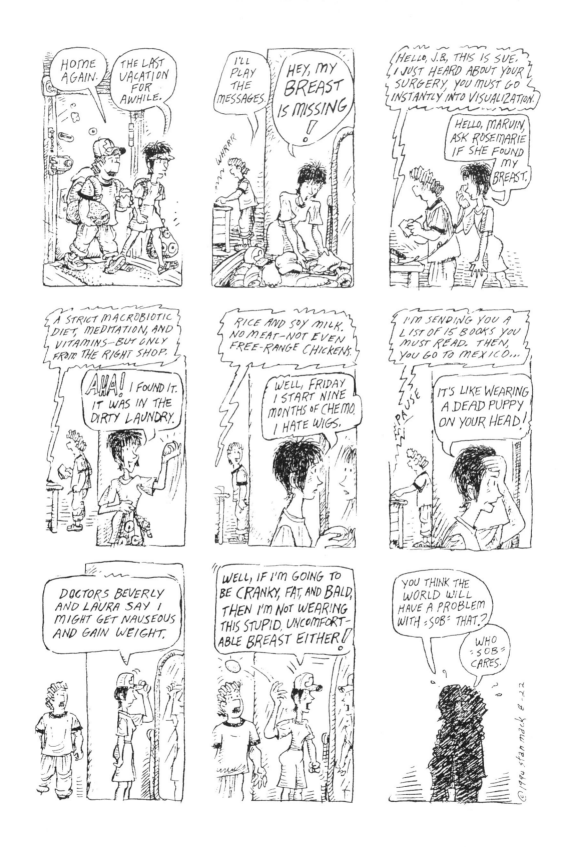

CHAPTER 2

Bring Your Own Chair

Janet was forced to make room in her life for cancer treatment.

Every three weeks she left her desk and traveled to the hospital to be measured, monitored, and infused with possibly life-saving but definitely toxic drugs.

The trip was a lengthy bus ride away. While the chemo made her tired, Janet was strong and liked to go by herself. She didn't feel like a patient and didn't want to be treated like one.

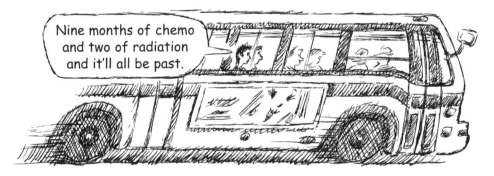

But I needed to be part of it, too. Half the time I'd go along, sitting by her side in the chemo suite, reading, schmoozing, joking. We had joined the community of people bound together by cancer.

The chemo suite was lined with chairs Janet called the blue Barcaloungers. In them sat the patients, some pale and wan, others seemingly healthy. They were tethered to plastic baggies containing various chemicals hanging from metal poles. The nurses moved among us, inserting and withdrawing needles, changing bags of medication, offering comfort and sweets.

Janet was naturally gregarious, but she also knew that being upbeat bought her more attention from the staff.

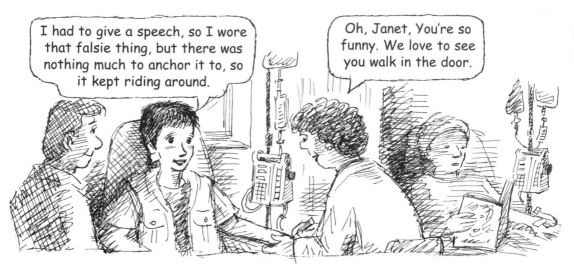

In those first few months, Janet was determined to maintain a sense of normalcy and control. And there was no doom in our words to each other.

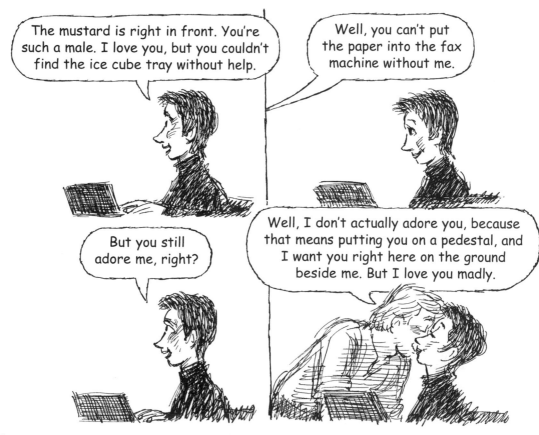

The cancer didn't change our love for each other. But some things were obviously different. How would I react to her having had a breast lopped off? Could I bring myself to touch her there? And should I? There was one thing I could be sure of—Janet wasn't going to hide in the dark.

Janet's hope (with her fingers crossed, I'm sure) was that I would still see her as the woman I wanted to make love to.

Full-body massages had always been a part of our lovemaking. The first few times after the surgery, I circled around her chest, avoiding the scarred part of her. But I didn't want to be like that. I wanted to live up to what I felt were her expectations of me.

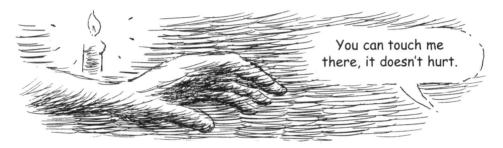

You can touch me there, it doesn't hurt.

It disturbed me at first. What was once smooth and soft was now puckered and unrecognizable. But, after a few attempts, I tentatively touched . . . and then gradually caressed her scar. I came to see that part of her as special, deserving tender attention.

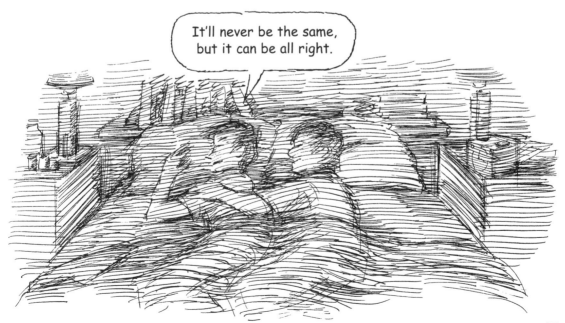

It'll never be the same, but it can be all right.

After a few rounds of chemo, her hair was falling out all over the apartment. Patches of scalp showed through and made her look sicker than she was. She said, "I think you'd better cut it all off." That weekend we visited a friend in Ocean City, Maryland. On her terrace overlooking the beach, I slowly cut away Janet's hair.

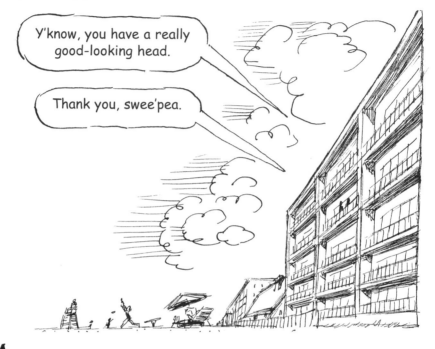

And then she was bald. Following the accepted wisdom in the breast cancer world, we went to buy a wig. But even during the fitting she was restless. For her, the wig was not a way to feel normal. It disguised who she was.

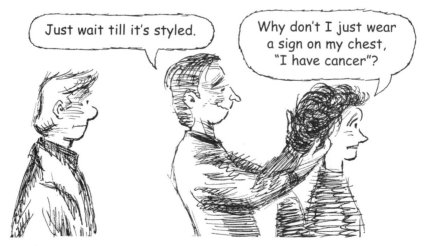

Carrying the boxed wig, we took the subway home. She counted three other bald people in our car. Two were women. "We live in Greenwich Village," she said, "where baldness is a fashion statement."

Back home, she tossed the wig in the closet.

Soon after, she wrote a letter to "Dear Abby." (Who among her sophisticated New York writer friends would ever write to an advice columnist?) To our amazement, they ran her letter.

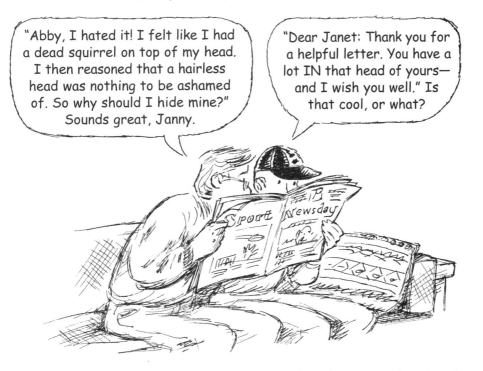

"Abby, I hated it! I felt like I had a dead squirrel on top of my head. I then reasoned that a hairless head was nothing to be ashamed of. So why should I hide mine?" Sounds great, Janny.

"Dear Janet: Thank you for a helpful letter. You have a lot IN that head of yours— and I wish you well." Is that cool, or what?

The only time Janet wore her wig was when she appeared on *Oprah* as an expert on teen violence. The production staff recommended that she wear her wig, because her baldness might distract from her topic. Janet agreed but was sorry afterwards because she hated how she looked.

We thought we knew what to expect in cancerland—the debilitating effects of chemo and radiation. But Janet's path also took some unexpected turns.

One morning, a third of the way through her chemotherapy, Janet woke up to find that the fingers of her right hand were twice their normal size and her right forearm was larger than her left.

She called her doctors, who said it was lymphedema, a swelling of the arm due to fluid buildup caused by the removal of lymph nodes. Because of the lack of lymph nodes, she would also be at a heightened risk of infection for the rest of her life. The main assistance they offered was mimeographed sheets of advice.

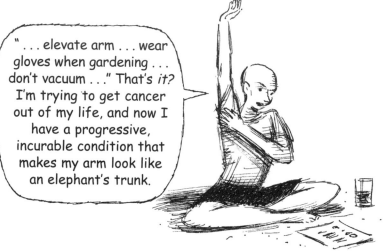

" . . . elevate arm . . . wear gloves when gardening . . . don't vacuum . . ." That's *it*? I'm trying to get cancer out of my life, and now I have a progressive, incurable condition that makes my arm look like an elephant's trunk.

She began to research the topic and discovered that two million to three million Americans, mostly women, suffered from lymphedema. She talked to several breast cancer patients and learned that their doctors dealt with the condition as though it were a minor and infrequent by-product of surgery.

She found her way to a smattering of health professionals around the country who specialized in treating lymphedema, sometimes competing for attention with the different treatment options. Her insurance company said that treatment was not reimbursable.

We determined that certain massage techniques were helpful, so I took that as my personal challenge. If I got it exactly, perfectly right, I could cure her arm. It was a little like gently squeezing a toothpaste tube.

Janet went to a seminar where they showed her how to wrap her arm nightly with three different kinds of compression bandages to keep the swelling down. So, from then on, I massaged and she wrapped.

In time, Janet discovered customized compression sleeves. Similar to compression stockings, the sleeves went from shoulder to hand. They proved very effective and she wore them all the time. She, of course, turned them into a fashion statement, black in the evening, blue during the day.

Along with her practical and methodical approach to her cancer, she joked to friends, "Dances around trees happily accepted."

Good-luck charms, protective amulets, and spiritual totems sent by well-wishers began to accumulate on our shelves.

Sally, an anthropologist and friend, who worked in the rain forests of western Africa, visited us. I did a comic strip on the day she and Janet went shopping for hats.

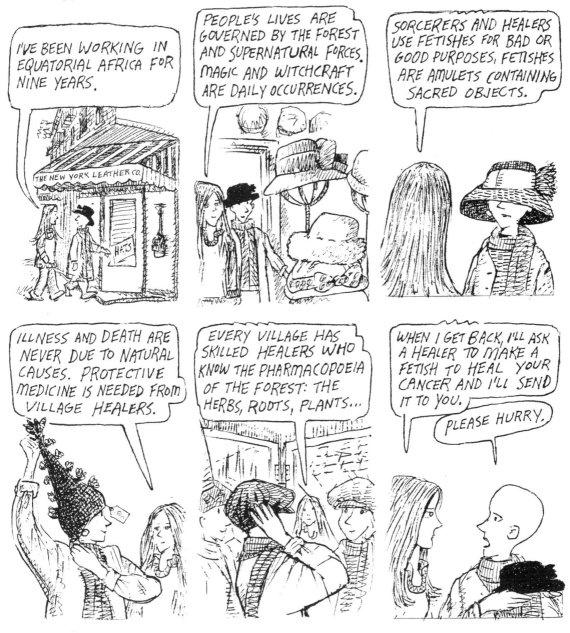

I'VE BEEN WORKING IN EQUATORIAL AFRICA FOR NINE YEARS.

THE NEW YORK LEATHER CO.

HATS

PEOPLE'S LIVES ARE GOVERNED BY THE FOREST AND SUPERNATURAL FORCES. MAGIC AND WITCHCRAFT ARE DAILY OCCURRENCES.

SORCERERS AND HEALERS USE FETISHES FOR BAD OR GOOD PURPOSES. FETISHES ARE AMULETS CONTAINING SACRED OBJECTS.

ILLNESS AND DEATH ARE NEVER DUE TO NATURAL CAUSES. PROTECTIVE MEDICINE IS NEEDED FROM VILLAGE HEALERS.

EVERY VILLAGE HAS SKILLED HEALERS WHO KNOW THE PHARMACOPOEIA OF THE FOREST: THE HERBS, ROOTS, PLANTS...

WHEN I GET BACK, I'LL ASK A HEALER TO MAKE A FETISH TO HEAL YOUR CANCER AND I'LL SEND IT TO YOU.

PLEASE HURRY.

Once back in Africa, Sally sent us a fetish made for Janet by a local medicine man. Though we could only guess what was in it, the fetish stood guard on Janet's bedside table.

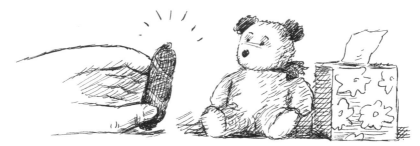

Strange growing fungi appeared on our kitchen counter. A friend had told us about a mushroom tea that he brewed and drank daily. He gave us cuttings from his mushrooms. We put them in jars of water where they grew as large as soup bowls and looked disgusting. Janet drank the tea every day for a year.

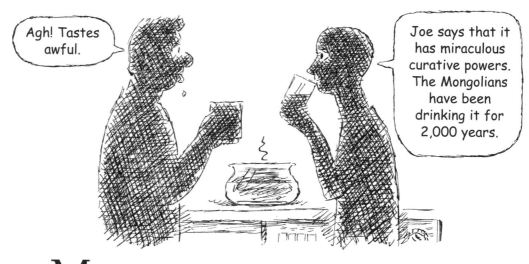

Meanwhile, she told herself that the destruction her body was going through was not as bad as problems other people faced. She used her illness as a way to connect with teens struggling with their own conflicts, and in the process, she comforted herself.

Agnes, a librarian for the New York Public Library for the Blind and Physically Handicapped, invited Janet to speak to the kids.

"Janet's book *Beating the Odds: Stories of Unexpected Achievers,* was in Braille and on cassette, so the kids knew her. On the day of her talk, a bald Janet faced a room full of kids with disabilities and said:

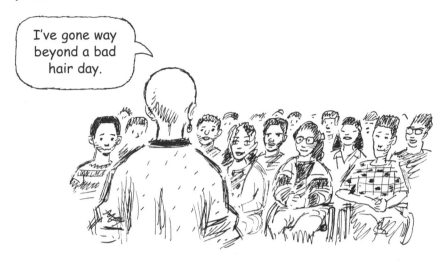

> I've gone way beyond a bad hair day.

"She opened up to them, told them about her cancer, let them feel her head, told them they weren't alone. Her face and body were so alive. She enjoyed the give and take of a live audience. She told them a cockroach story that grossed me out and that they loved. Afterwards, the kids ignored their snack and their buses and stayed and talked to her. One kid, with every disability in the book, said:

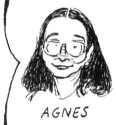

AGNES

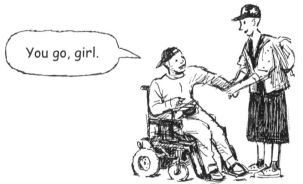

> You go, girl.

"I was losing most of my own sight by then. I was angry at everyone including my wonderful husband, but I couldn't talk about it. When Janet finished, I thought, if she can do it, I can. I went home and said to my husband, 'You're my salvation, I'm your penance.' And our laughter dried my tears."

Though she was sick from the chemo, she also accepted an invitation to speak to juvenile offenders at a maximum security facility in Oregon. Freeda was the facility staff person who set up the appearance.

"Most of these kids are dysfunctional and violent and like to wallow in self-pity. My job is to try to give them some hope by bringing in interesting speakers.

"When Janet and Stan arrived, we marched the kids to the auditorium and seated them under heavy guard. They looked bored. Who cared about a middle-aged woman even if she was wearing a polka-dot baseball cap?

"Janet talked about the kids she'd interviewed who were struggling with drugs, gang violence, and of the ones who had the courage to overcome their problems. Then she took a step closer to the first row and pulled off her baseball cap to reveal her bald head. It was as though an electrical charge shot through the room and Janet had their full attention."

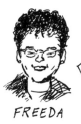

FREEDA

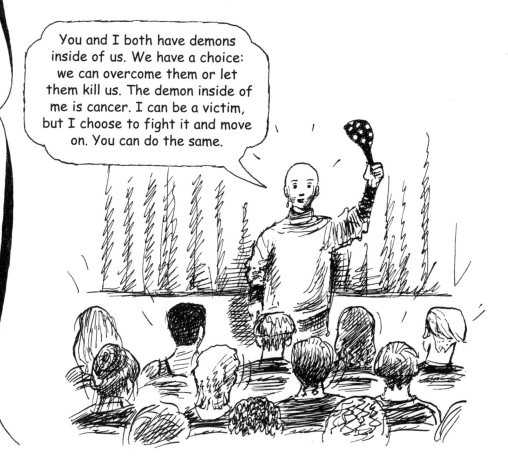

You and I both have demons inside of us. We have a choice: we can overcome them or let them kill us. The demon inside of me is cancer. I can be a victim, but I choose to fight it and move on. You can do the same.

Meanwhile, she began battling another kind of cancer, this time human-made, one which humans could cure but won't. As the treatment progressed, Janet became entangled in billing hell.

In her first meetings with her doctors, Beverly and Laura, Janet tried to anticipate reimbursement problems by making sure her doctors were on her insurance plan. "Janet," Laura said, "even though their rates are terrible, I've joined your HMO so you'll be covered."

Janet assumed that because her oncologist was covered, the cancer center where her oncologist practiced would also be covered. Wrong! Manhattan Hospital itself had no relationship with her HMO, causing Janet acute and unnecessary stress. For example, some months into chemo, we discovered that the insurance company was paying for the chemicals but rejecting the facility charge—in effect, denying the chair that Janet sat in.

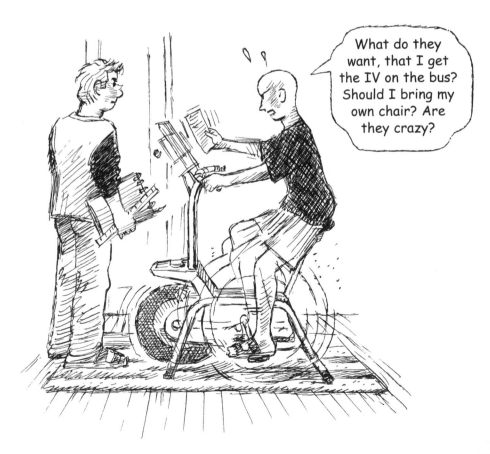

The facility and other unpaid charges piled up and were automatically sent to a collection agency, which then harassed Janet—who couldn't figure out what she was being billed for. She spent hours on the phone and in person with the hospital's billing people trying to unravel the mystery.

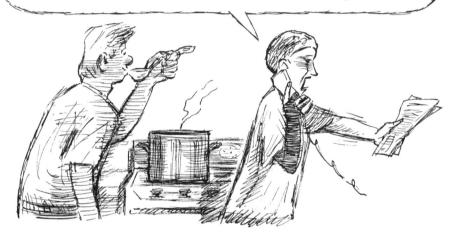

I'm trying to understand what this late charge is for. Meanwhile, your collection agency keeps threatening me—even though Florence promised me you wouldn't put it into collection. What do you mean, you're Florence and we've never talked before? The doctors are trying to save me while you guys in billing are trying to kill me!

The funny thing was, Janet's combination of outrage and empathy often turned foes into allies.

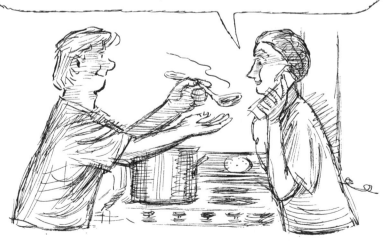

Florence, darling, it's not you. I know you're only doing your job. I'm sure you're overworked and underpaid. It's your child's first week at day care? That can be so difficult.

No matter how friendly she was, Janet knew to keep a complete and chronological dossier of her hospital bills and HMO statements. She took notes on every conversation, including first and last names. As the charges piled up, she moved from clerks to supervisors to department heads and finally in frustration she took it all the way to the state insurance board.

Janet had finally gotten their attention. It was to take two years, but a meeting was held between the director of patient accounts, the assistant director of outpatient billing, and the hospital's ombudsman on one side and Janet on the other. The result was that they gave Janet a dollar amount she felt was reasonable. There would be no confusion this time. Janet's tape recorder sat in the middle of the table.

In the meantime, too late to help Janet, her insurance company changed its policy and began to cover the outpatient facility charge.

In July '95, one year after entering cancerland, Janet's chemo and radiation came to an end. It was sort of anticlimactic. No diploma, no gold watch. Just "Okay, you're done."

But by then Janet's hair had begun to grow back. And it was coming in wavy, something she'd always wanted!

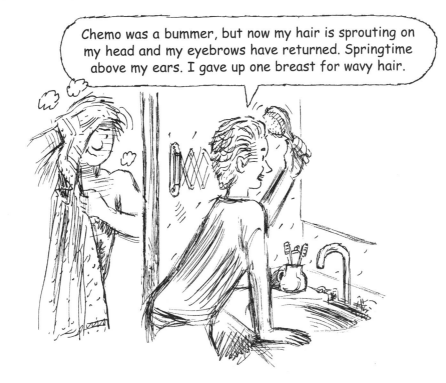

35

The same week, *The Village Voice*, where for twenty years I had produced a weekly comic strip, suddenly and unceremoniously dumped a number of features, including my strip. Being cut loose that way was a blow to my self-esteem and my wallet. But there was a silver lining. For the first time in twenty years, I didn't have a weekly deadline.

Coincidently, Janet and I received good professional news. Our latest manuscript—a book on teens in prison—was accepted for publication, and we were paid the last half of the advance.

For Janet, all this added up to only one thing: we were free to celebrate her release from cancer treatment by living out a dream of ours. We would circle the globe.

We decided to hit the road on a six-week trip, starting in Tahiti and working our way west.

She passed a blood test and we got our shots. We found a guy in a little travel shop who altered Janet's backpack so that its weight hung only from her good shoulder. And we packed for the trip in our usual way. Whatever didn't fit into our packs didn't go.

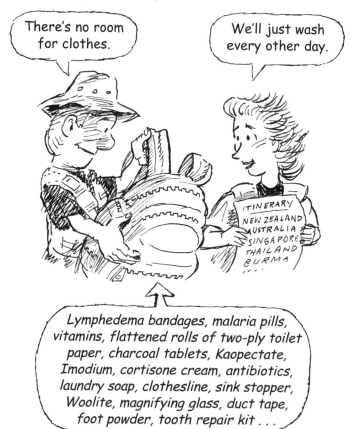

We left on September 11, 1995.

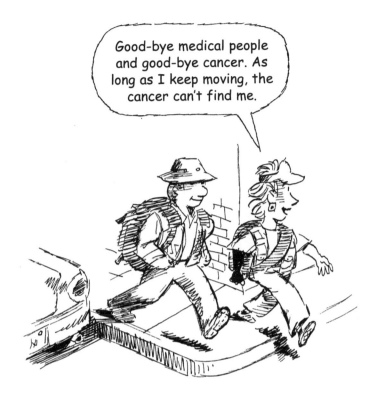

CHAPTER 3

Love in the Afternoon

Our round-the-world adventure took us to the red desert of Australia, high tea at Raffles in Singapore, the Buddhist temples of Burma. . . .

Janet and I had always traveled on our own to distant, often offbeat, sometimes risky destinations, entirely dependent on each other, and loving every moment.

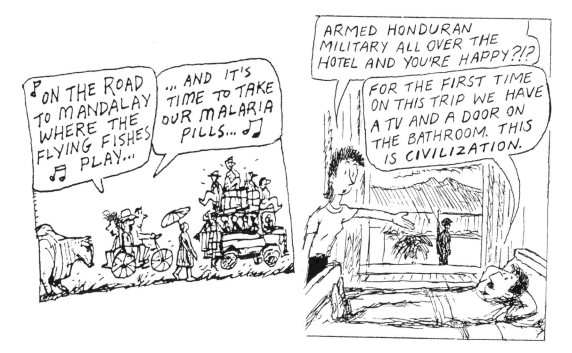

I thought about how well we fit together and yet how unlikely it was that she and I had found each other at all.

In the early '70s, I was married, had two nice kids, and lived in the suburbs. I'd been an art director at *The New York Times* and left to become a freelance humorous illustrator for magazines and children's books. Life was good, but I was restless.

New York was caught in the social, political, sexual, and artistic upheavals of the day, and the vibrations were rattling my cage. I came up with an idea that would put me in the middle of the action: a documentary-style comic strip covering the New York scene.

Part cub reporter, part voyeur, part vagabond, I wandered the city in search of the mad or meaningful. I learned to blend into places I didn't belong and take notes on my shirt cuff. I wrote down what people said, sketched them saying it, and turned my notes into a new kind of cartoon journalism. The strip ran in *The Village Voice*, the leading counterculture weekly of the day, beginning in late '74.

I don't know whether I created the strip because I was going through a midlife crisis or whether the strip created the crisis, but *Stan Mack's Real Life Funnies* changed the direction of my career and my life.

Every week I left my house, stepping over the kids' bikes in the driveway, and went to town. I became a believer at a UFO convention, a protestor at an anti-nuke demonstration, a bachelor at a singles' rap session, a dildo salesman at the Pink Pussycat Boutique. . . .

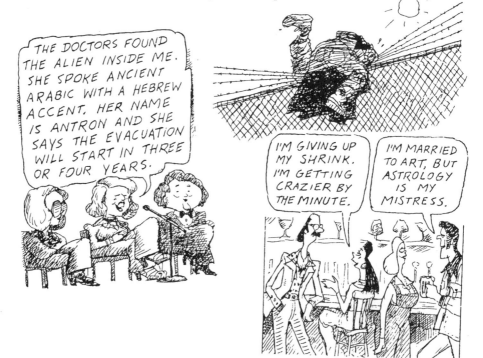

As my strips grew in notoriety and took more and more of my time, my marriage grew rockier.

One day in 1980 the *Voice* ran an ad for a bisexual conference to be held in Greenwich Village—perfect grist for me. I told an editor at the *Voice* that I planned to go. He asked me to meet a freelance writer named Janet Bode at the door and give her a *Voice* press pass.

I remember what Janet looked like that day: jeans tucked into Frye boots, close-fitting brown blazer, Joan Baez hair, slim, about five feet five, flashing eyes, and one earring.

After the conference we went for a beer. She was magnetic. I thought she might be a story for my strip. Instead we gabbed for hours about our work and our lives. She was fascinated by what I did, as I was by what she revealed about her past.

She'd recently arrived in New York after ten years in the sex, drugs, and rock 'n' roll world of San Francisco where she'd been part of the scene, done local reporting, and even written a book on rape. But, she said, to further her writing career, she had to be in New York. With few contacts, she picked up and came east with her new boyfriend Howie, a sweet guy, cross-country trucker, and closet heroin addict.

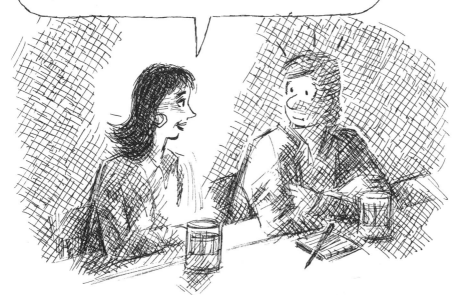

When I found out, I tried to help him get clean . . . I'd even plead with him from the back of his Harley when he went to cop drugs but finally had to leave him . . . I turned the whole thing into an article for *New York* magazine . . . he's now in rehab and we're still friends.

Her enthusiasm, curiosity about people, and love of a good story were contagious. In the following weeks I'd sometimes pick her up to come along on my comic strip forays.

In June of '81, Janet invited me to join her when she went to Fire Island to help write a humorous, soft-core musical. Funny sex talk? Of course I went.

That afternoon Janet and I took a walk on the beach. She wasn't trying to be seductive, and I didn't intend to flirt, but somehow we got to holding hands.

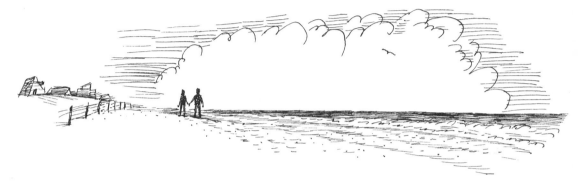

After that I avoided her. I thought of her as a buddy, and I wasn't in the market anyway. Then one day we bumped into each other at the *Voice,* and she told me a funny conversation she'd had with a cab driver, which I turned into a strip. I realized again how much we thought alike.

Later that afternoon, back at her apartment, we made love—after I first poked her in the eye with my elbow. So cool.

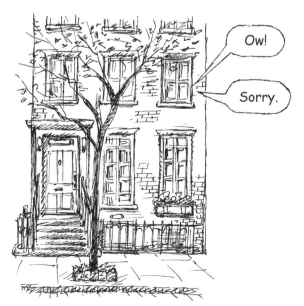

We began a fling—not forever, just for now. Part of my New York fantasy life, and maybe hers. Soon we were meeting secretly and regularly. We'd fool around, then sit on her bed trading ideas and reading each other's work. The fling became an affair. I was full of guilt about my family. Janet felt guilty about adding to another woman's pain. Yet neither of us would end it.

Janet's close friends gradually found out about us and worried about her.

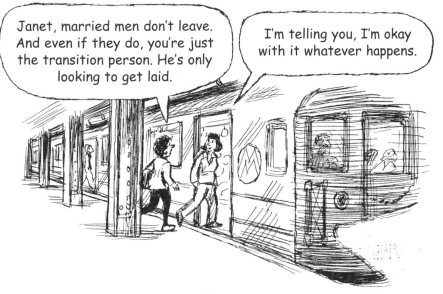

One of her friends, Jim, who'd known her in San Francisco, had a different view.

"Crazy guys with their own hang-ups were her thing. Stan was nice to her and the only mature relationship she'd ever had."

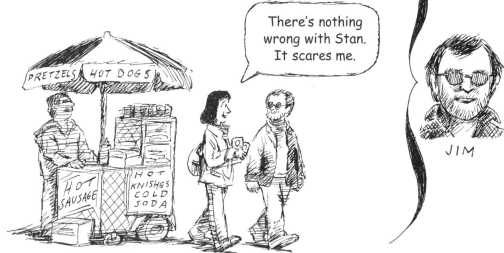

43

I was a little nervous, too—for different reasons.

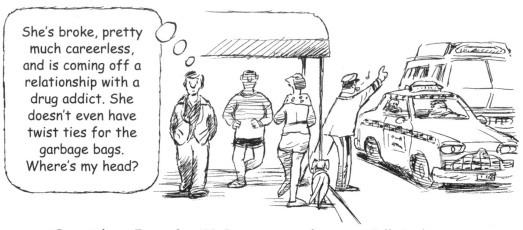

She's broke, pretty much careerless, and is coming off a relationship with a drug addict. She doesn't even have twist ties for the garbage bags. Where's my head?

One night in December '82, Janet went with me to a Billy Joel concert on Long Island. I was doing a comic strip from backstage. Janet sat in the audience. Afterwards I couldn't find her. I knew she could get home, but I was suddenly seized by a deep sense of loss so intense it shocked me. We finally met up, but I realized this was way more than an affair.

One doesn't audition for jumping off a cliff. After months of stress and indecision, I just did it. I told her I was her birthday present and showed up at her door with some art supplies, my bedboard for my bad back, and a handful of twist ties. I don't think either of us expected me to do it.

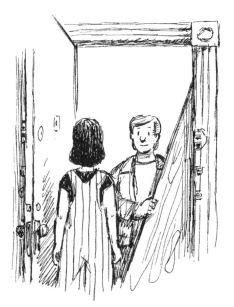

For the next year or so we had bumpy times. Janet was stressed trying to become a writer and make ends meet. My two teenage sons withdrew in a tangle of confused feelings. It would be a few years before they used our apartment as a convenient city stop-off and Janet as a worldly advisor. At first, I was spending so much time in the suburbs with my kids that Janet accused me of dating my wife. But we made a pact to try never to go to bed mad.

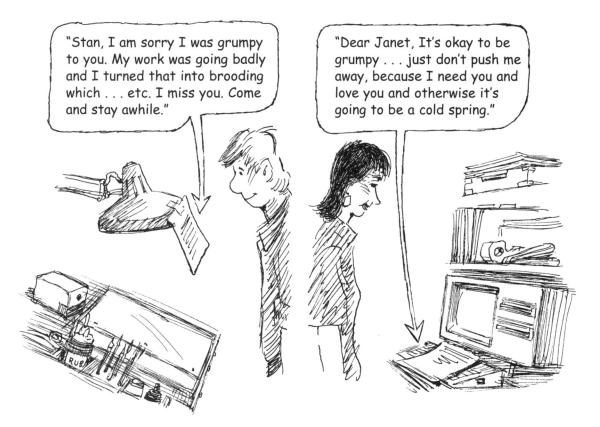

Unconventional as our beginning may have been, Janet and I did get the approval of two of the most important people in our lives—her sister Carolyn and my mother—despite their initial misgivings.

"We were all shocked that Janet, my independent sister, and Stan were together so much. I couldn't believe she wasn't feeling smothered. I'd been suspicious of him, but when we met, I saw he was smitten by her. I began to think they might make it."

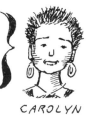

CAROLYN

45

At the end of our first year, Janet and I drove to Providence and I introduced her to my mom. My mother had taped a picture of my ex-wife on the refrigerator and was prepared to disapprove of this shiksa her son had taken up with. But in a short time she came to love Janet and assumed any accomplishment of mine was Janet's doing.

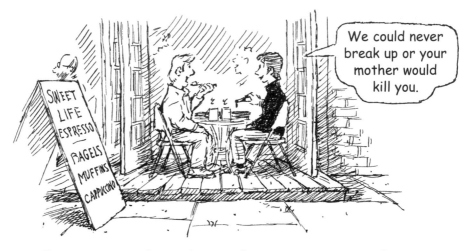

Our new partnership took many shapes, some unexpected.

I became her hairdresser—though my main experience had been trimming the yew bushes around my house. I turned her long, straight, thin hair into a short, spiky cut that she loved. Along with her single earring, it became her look.

She introduced me to the world. My only foreign travel had been a trip to Paris. Now, yearly, we hit the road with our packs and my little fold-up back seat and headed for exotic places like Petra in Jordan and Tikal in Guatemala.

Eleven years after I showed up with my bedboard and twist ties, we'd become best friends, lovers, travel partners, and professional collaborators. She'd found her way to an important career writing hard-hitting nonfiction books for and about teenagers. We worked side by side in our loft. We traded ideas in the shower, edited each other's pictures and words over beers, and often went along on each other's assignments.

We also went about our mundane tasks, like laundry every Saturday morning, with breakfast at the corner diner between the wash and dry cycles. We'd order eggs, I'd eat the whites, she'd eat my yolks. We'd joke about how underappreciated our work was and how it was a good thing we appreciated each other.

I made elaborate and silly birthday cards for her.

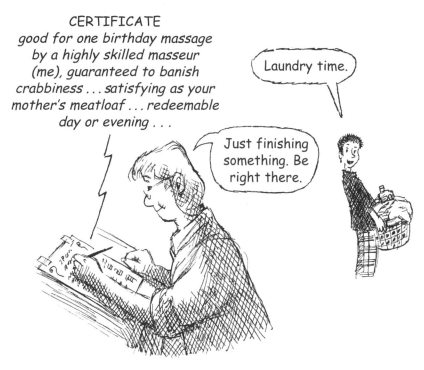

CERTIFICATE
*good for one birthday massage
by a highly skilled masseur
(me), guaranteed to banish
crabbiness . . . satisfying as your
mother's meatloaf . . . redeemable
day or evening . . .*

Laundry time.

Just finishing something. Be right there.

Janet expressed her appreciation for me to Carolyn in her typically direct way.

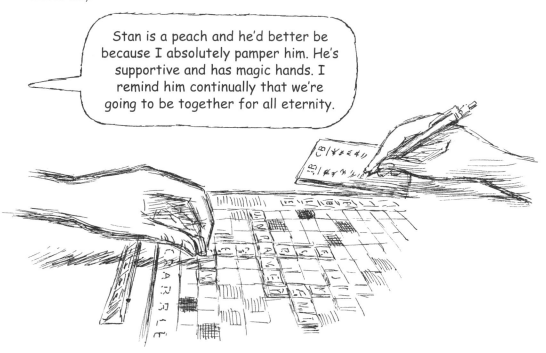

Stan is a peach and he'd better be because I absolutely pamper him. He's supportive and has magic hands. I remind him continually that we're going to be together for all eternity.

Then she felt a lump in her breast.

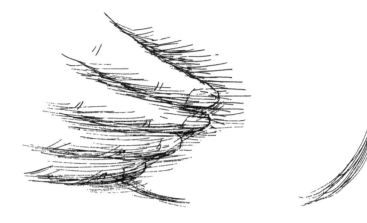

CHAPTER 4

The Best of Times

Janet had made it through the year of diagnosis, mastectomy, chemo, and radiation. And then she reclaimed her old self with our trip around the world. Late in October of '95, tired and happy, we returned home, ready to renew our pre-cancer life.

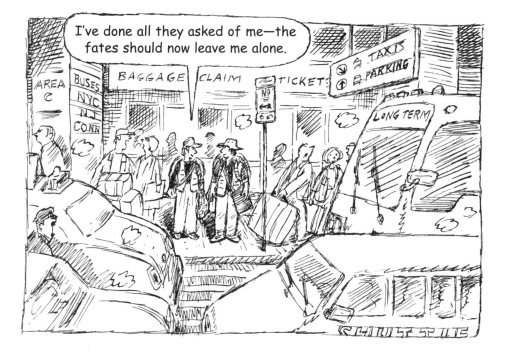

Friends would refer to Janet as being in remission. She and I never used that word. It suggested that the cancer might be lying hidden, waiting to jump out and attack again. It was a word for defeatists. Janet was cancer free.

For the next three years, Janet kept up her energetic schedule of writing, speaking at schools around the country, and appearing as a teen expert on radio and TV. During that time, I began a major book project of my own, a history of the Jewish people illustrated with my cartoons. It would be an attempt to reclaim my own roots.

Janet visited Carolyn in Los Angeles and said to her:

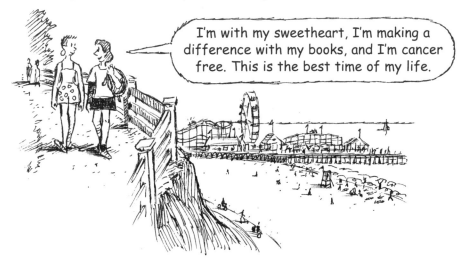

I'm with my sweetheart, I'm making a difference with my books, and I'm cancer free. This is the best time of my life.

From time to time, anxiety about her health would grip me, but my role was clear; support her in her conviction that she'd beaten the cancer.

Our days took on the look and feel they'd had before her illness, except that she would sometimes lie on the couch reading the paper and complain of a lack of energy.

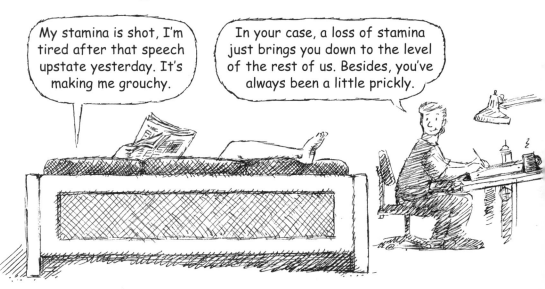

My stamina is shot, I'm tired after that speech upstate yesterday. It's making me grouchy.

In your case, a loss of stamina just brings you down to the level of the rest of us. Besides, you've always been a little prickly.

By the third year after the end of the treatment, we were gaining confidence that the disease was really gone. Laura's words—that the more pessimistic statistics were ten years old and that lots of women in Janet's category were doing well—resonated in my head.

But Janet had misgivings. She spoke of them with her friend Kathryn, the fourth member of Janet's writers' group to be diagnosed with cancer. In their e-mails to each other, Janet revealed details she didn't always share with me.

Kathryn, I don't know which aches are treatment induced and which are old age. When I'm walking, I feel like I have no padding on the bottom of my feet, and my bones feel brittle and battered.

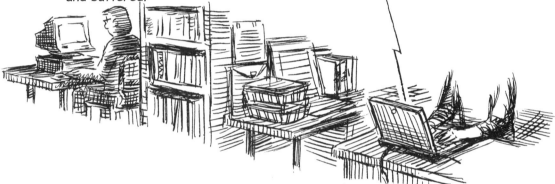

And they both complained about "chemo brain."

Kathryn, I seem to be losing my memory—especially my visual memory. Today I didn't recognize a neighbor and Stan made the excuse that I didn't have my glasses.

Janet, I know all about chemo brain. Doctors say to me, "You look great, tests are fine." They don't talk about the near-empty cavity in my head that once was my brain and now holds a small walnut.

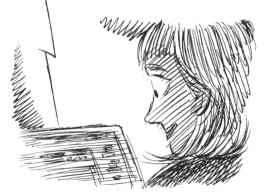

Even as Janet continued to be monitored by her doctors, she and Kathryn spoke about crossing a line that put them in the "shadow of death."

Kathryn, am I in denial about cancer because I postpone tests, or is it that I'm tired of tests that give inconclusive results: "Something on the X-ray . . . need more tests . . . oops, nothing there . . . sorry." I just want to go on blissfully unaware and then be struck dead.

Janet, tests don't cause cancer. I'm glad you went.

Kathryn, I had a dream last night. A not particularly threatening bearded man was coming towards me on the sidewalk. He had a gun and, as we passed, I wondered if he was going to use it. He did. He shot me in the back.

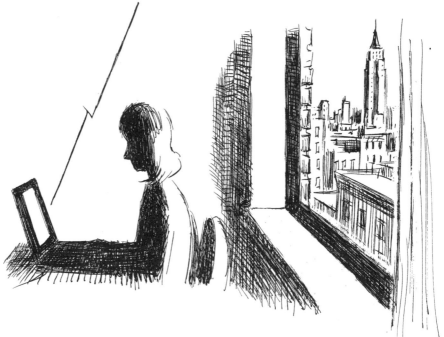

In the summer of '98, I finally delivered my historical opus—four thousand years of the Jewish experience. Janet had recently handed in her most ambitious book, *Colors of Freedom*, a look at the immigrant experience, with oral histories, poems, recipes, and kids' drawings—scheduled to be published in the fall of '99. She was bone-tired and we both longed to get out from behind our desks and go far away.

We had a picture calendar hanging on our kitchen wall. It showed the mysterious Inca ruins of Machu Picchu, high up in the Peruvian Andes, said to be a global center of spirituality and healing. Janet always dreamed of making that journey.

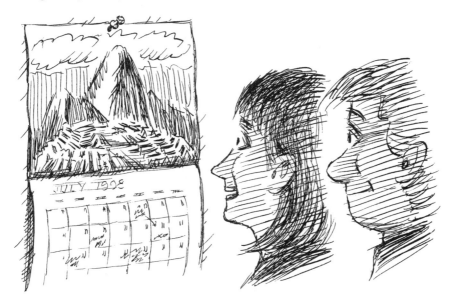

I knew she'd slowed a bit since her year of treatment, but I also knew she was never happier than when she was on the road. We decided to fly to Ecuador and sail the Galápagos Islands, and then visit Machu Picchu.

If my calculations are correct, we're going to be at Machu Picchu during the full moon.

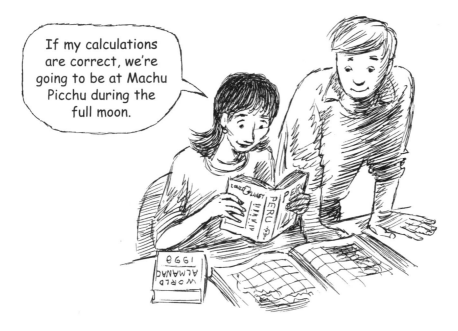

Janet e-mailed Kathryn once more:

I have to go on this trip. I'm feeling a sense of urgency that I don't want to go into with Stan. If the situation were reversed, I probably wouldn't want to listen to his whining about how he might die any minute.

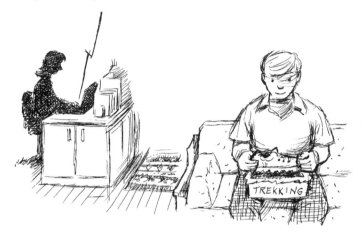

We left in August—once more doing what Janet loved so much. And, as usual, her spirit lifted and carried me aloft.

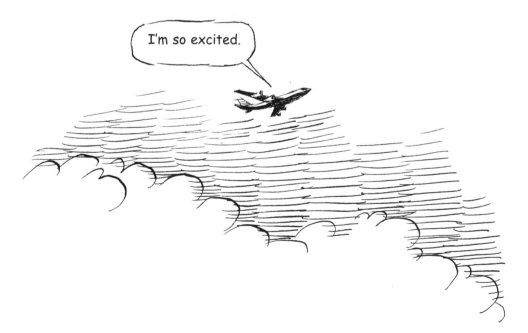

CHAPTER 5

Indeterminate Focal Abnormality

For a week, we cruised the Galápagos Islands off the coast of Ecuador. We explored lava cliffs, stood toe to webbed toe with blue-footed boobies, and laughingly tried to make love in our tiny cabin.

From sea level, by plane and switchback train, we made our way up to Machu Picchu. In that mystical place, we hiked paths the ancient Incas walked, and I took pictures of her with her big smile and arms thrown into the air.

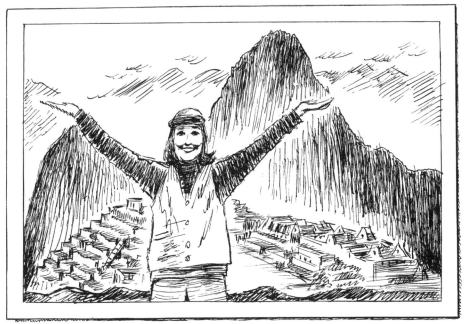

But she began to complain of chest pain, which we assumed was strain brought on by breathing the thinner air.

Back home, Laura sent her for tests. Janet had been cancer free for almost exactly three years. A week after the tests, Laura reported that Janet's cancer was back.

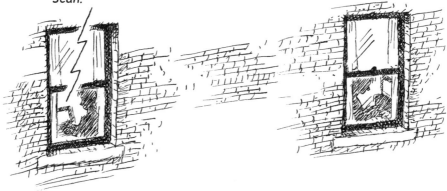

IMPRESSION:

Abnormal scintigraphic activity correspon to one-half of the sternum which corresp the plain film radiographs, findings osseous metastatic lesion.

Indeterminate focal abnormality involving for which there is no plain film radiog time. Finding is suggestive of, but not di of metastasis.

Diffusely increased activity associat... posteriorly which may be asso...: pleural effusion an...

The news was a shock that Janet and I faced in different ways. I am into avoidance. I put the news in a box labeled "open only if forced." Otherwise I followed her lead. She, on the other hand, quickly decided that she would beat it again. She added the treatment schedule to her crowded calendar and went back to work.

Janet, who never wanted to write about cancer but was a natural reporter, wasn't shy about discussing her cancer's return in e-mails to and meetings with friends, often using a flip humor that made her seem in control.

Laura said the bone scan showed "an abnormality in the lower portion of the sternum that appears to be consistent with the breast disease." She reminded me that my tumor was very aggressive. I said it might be peanut butter on the scan.

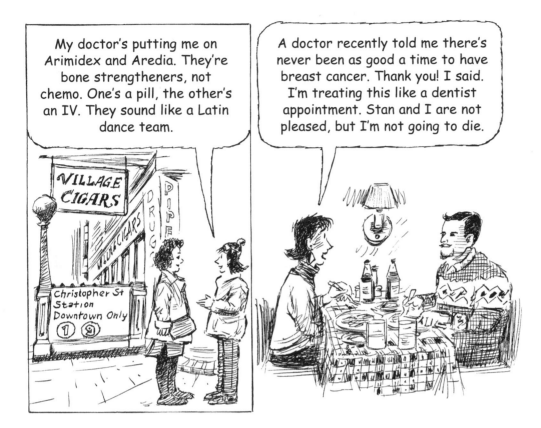

My doctor's putting me on Arimidex and Aredia. They're bone strengtheners, not chemo. One's a pill, the other's an IV. They sound like a Latin dance team.

A doctor recently told me there's never been as good a time to have breast cancer. Thank you! I said. I'm treating this like a dentist appointment. Stan and I are not pleased, but I'm not going to die.

In the early stages of the return, Janet's spirit and energy were fine. She was working on a new book. And we did a three-state swing through the West where we interviewed teens and Janet spoke to them.

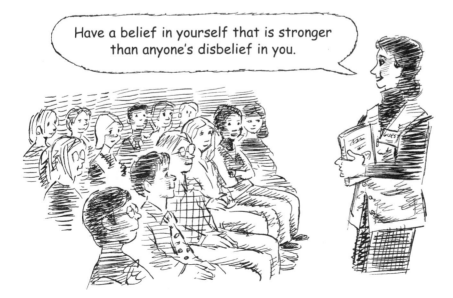

Have a belief in yourself that is stronger than anyone's disbelief in you.

In the winter she felt draggy and developed a cough. She had all the signs of a typical New York City cold. She took heavy-duty antibiotics, but they gave her no relief. To top it off, she developed painful mouth sores, one result of her weakened immune system. She said, "I'm basically fine—just a little pooped."

In February I suggested a vacation to the Florida Keys to bake out the cold.

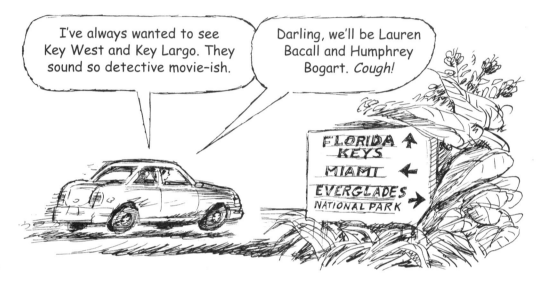

We stayed at the Proud Pelican in Key Largo and joined the wharf rats watching the sunset at Key West. But Janet continued to feel tired and would ask that I bring dinner back to the motel. In the past, Janet's positive energy had always swept me along like a big wave. Now I felt the first cold touch of fear—that this time the disease could really hurt her.

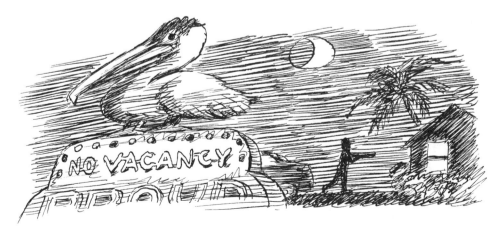

She returned to New York with the same lethargy and cough, and new bone pain. Laura scheduled her for a battery of tests.

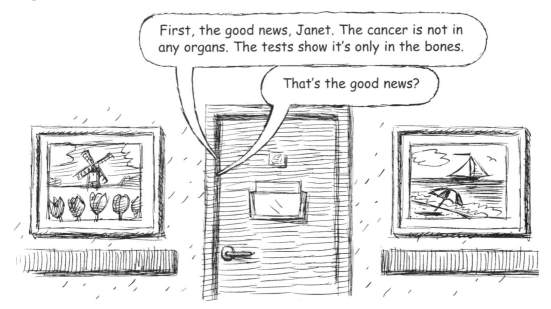

> The MRI was fun since I'm claustrophobic. They gave me a tranquilizer breakfast and handed me a blindfold. Still, I screamed in harmony with the machine.

> YEOWWW

On March 14, 1999, we bused over to the hospital to meet Laura and get the results of the tests.

> First, the good news, Janet. The cancer is not in any organs. The tests show it's only in the bones.

> That's the good news?

Then she said, "Now the bad news. The treatment you've been on for six months isn't working. The cancer has spread to your left arm, left leg, skull, spine, and pelvis. It's too diffuse for radiation so we'll schedule chemo, which will treat all the areas at once."

The word *skull* really shook me. I looked over at Janet. She looked Laura in the eye . . . and asked for the truth.

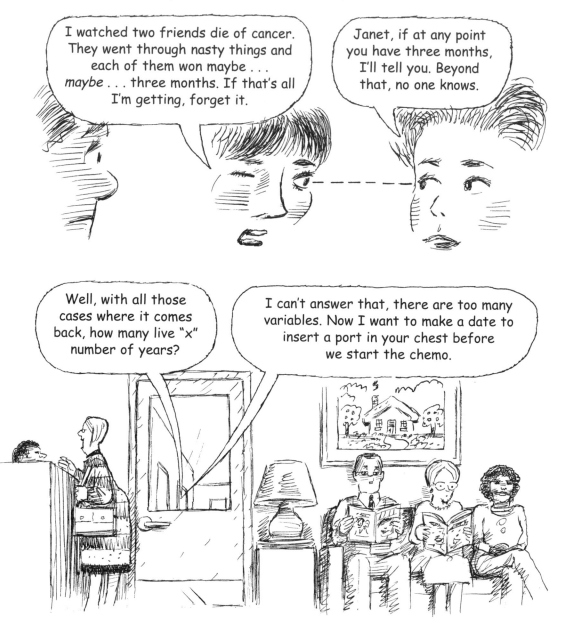

I watched two friends die of cancer. They went through nasty things and each of them won maybe . . . *maybe* . . . three months. If that's all I'm getting, forget it.

Janet, if at any point you have three months, I'll tell you. Beyond that, no one knows.

Well, with all those cases where it comes back, how many live "x" number of years?

I can't answer that, there are too many variables. Now I want to make a date to insert a port in your chest before we start the chemo.

Port. We were back in cancerland and speaking its language.

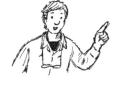

Port: a catheter inserted under the skin just below the collarbone. Through it the chemo nurse can draw blood and inject chemicals.

Janet needed the port because of the lymphedema in her right arm. The nurse could only insert the IV in her left hand and, as a result, her veins had begun to collapse. Physically, the port was much better for Janet. Symbolically, it was worse—she was now a permanent patient.

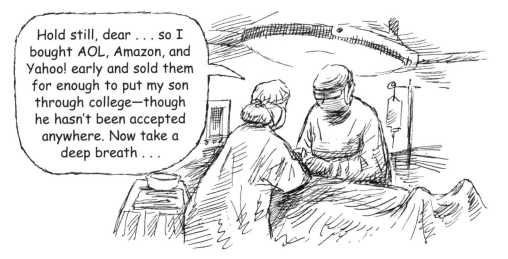

Laura scheduled a chemo drug cocktail of Taxol and Herceptin, with a side order of steroids.

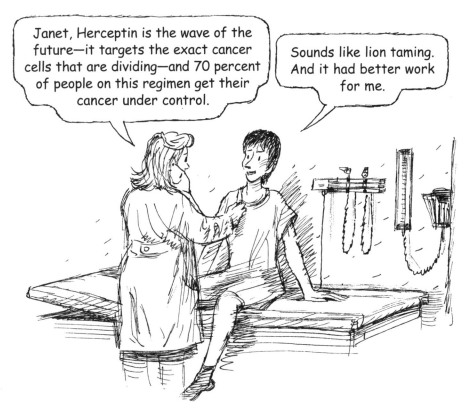

There were always friends who urged Janet to get second opinions, but Janet had made a decision to stay with Laura. She liked her personally and she trusted her medical judgment. In addition to her regular checkups, Janet and Laura kept up regular e-mail correspondence. Laura said it was easier for her to communicate that way. And it allowed Janet to send health updates.

Laura, I just finished this week's chemo and radiation, pain lessening, went on a twenty-minute walk to 14th Street. I no longer feel like eating small children.

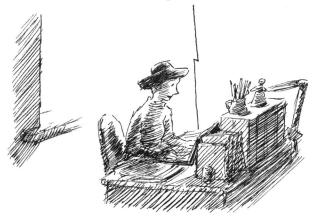

With the promise of Herceptin, we found a way to be optimistic. I pictured her bones with clustered dots of cancer, and the Herceptin like little Pacmen gobbling them one by one.

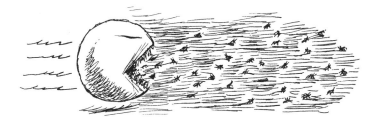

At first, with the chemo and steroids and pain medication, she began to feel better.

Janet was confident that she was still in charge of her fate, but we were now embarked on an emotional and physical roller-coaster. My job was to assure her that I was okay and we were okay.

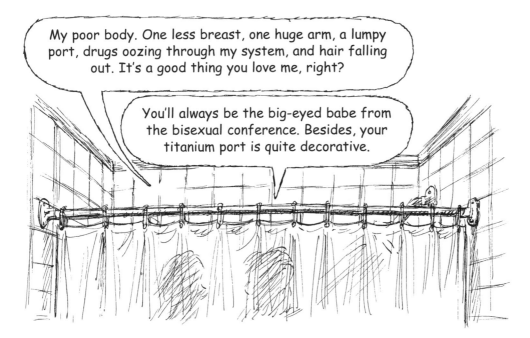

The chemo left her bald once again. It sapped her energy but didn't blunt her tongue.

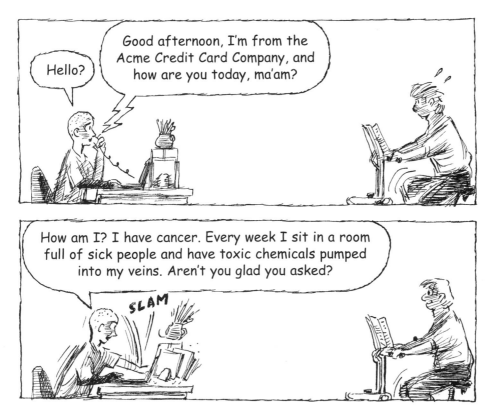

During May, Janet's physical problems worsened: bone pain, nosebleeds, tingling fingers, ringing ears. She continued trying to incorporate the treatment into her life. She edited her manuscript while getting chemo—working faster when the steroids kicked in, slowing down with the Benadryl.

And she had her first blood transfusion. It gave her renewed energy, and she spoke at a conference of young-adult librarians in Florida with someone else's blood zipping through her veins.

Back home, she found it harder to walk, but she rode her desk like a fighter pilot, shooting out e-mails. She talked of dying, but she didn't really believe it.

The hospital is adding a surcharge to medical bills—sure, take advantage of sick people! I called my state assembly guy and said he better do something about this before I die.

Just got off the phone from ranting at my editor. Now feeling pretty good. Better than worrying about blood markers.

Angry at a dear friend who tells me the way to beat breast cancer is to have a good attitude. Like if I die, I wasn't optimistic enough? Fit her for cement shoes.

This was a lousy day where I screamed in self-pity and suggested to Stan that he might want to go to New Jersey to escape my wrath. And he considered it!!!

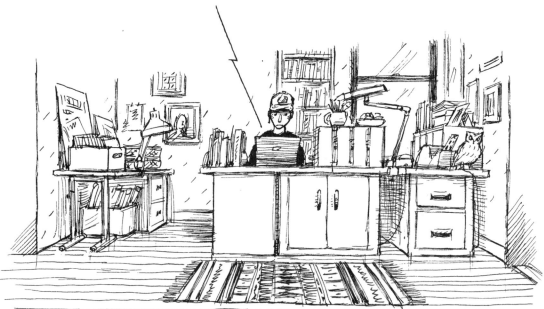

Janet's week was filling up with heart tests and bone scans and chemo visits and nap breaks and the compiling of a pain diary and medication schedule and the organizing of her growing and colorful array of pills.

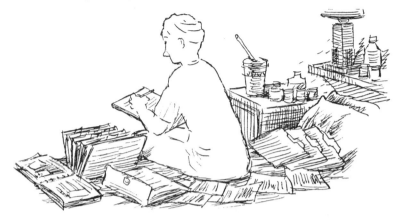

Without at first realizing it, I was, by myself, doing more of our little everyday tasks—shopping, laundry, dishes. One day while I was leaning over the sink, it hit me why my back was beginning to pain me.

My whole life I'd never used a dishwasher, but now I found myself buying a newer one from a neighbor and using it every day. Make way for Kitchen Man!

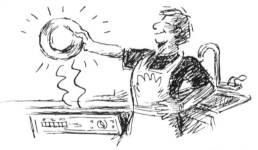

Janet's wisecracks disguised the seriousness of her disease for many, but some knew better. One night, our friends Liz and Richard came over with a pot of jambalaya, the first of many dinners they'd deliver over the next several months.

"Janet was funny talking about her treatment, but it sounded to me like a virulent form of the cancer and she was looking drawn. Stan had said Janet was losing interest in eating. He wasn't looking so robust himself. I decided to cook for Janet. I'm a control freak. I said to Richard, 'If I can keep feeding her, we can hold on to her.'"

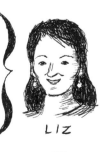

LIZ

When they arrived that first night, I was surprised to discover that it bothered me. Did it mean I wasn't taking proper care of the two of us? Did they think Janet was an invalid? It made me aware that our friends were talking about us.

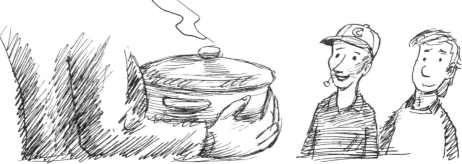

Janet and I had also begun nighttime phone conversations with an old friend, Kate, a midwife at a big Boston hospital. Kate, an avid kayaker, would call us late at night from her apartment, or her van, or from some remote riverside camp. She offered us medical insight—and her incredible heart.

"Janet's questions were always about content, like bone issues and treatment options. Stan's questions were about process, like what to do about her diet. I knew some big-shot doctors at my hospital and I'd chase them for answers. I'd call one oncologist at home and talk to him over the sounds of his baby splashing in the tub. He said Herceptin worked with some people, but that given Janet's tumor nature, everything else looked bad.

"It seemed to me that Janet's health was going downhill. But Janet and Stan didn't want to hear that. I told them about a friend who was still around twelve years after metastasis to the sternum."

KATE

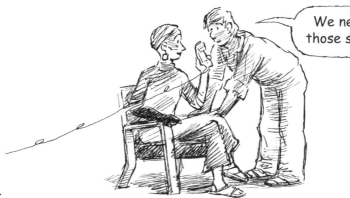

We need more of those stories, Kate.

Gradually Janet talked to Kate less. But, night after night, as Janet slept, I would talk to Kate, walking her through our days, and her voice coming into our apartment was my lifeline.

Often now, when I'd give updates on Janet's condition, I would suddenly get teary and not be able to finish sentences. I discovered that if I ran my wrists under cold water, it cooled me down and turned off the tears. Kate got so used to it that when she heard a certain catch in my voice, she'd say:

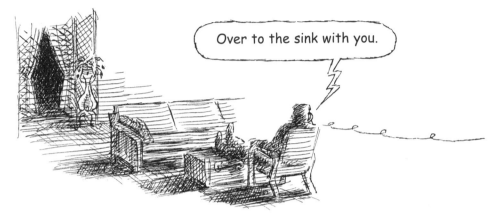

By June, Janet was knee-deep in chemo. For a time she thought she could expend greater effort and keep up with her normal schedule. She'd deflect questions from publishing people by joking that yes, she was in breast cancer treatment—wasn't everyone? But now she was really struggling and beginning to move like an old lady.

Then Janet and I went in to see Laura for one of her regular checkups. And we heard that Janet would never again be cancer free.

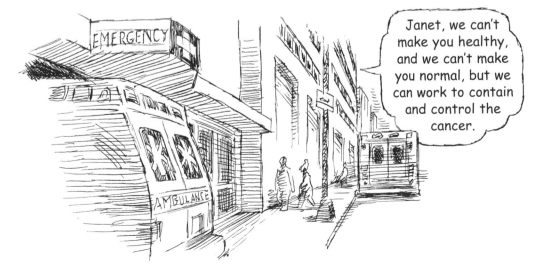

Janet and I always felt our spirits rise when we stood on a beach looking out across the water. Now we headed for the walkway along the Hudson River, leaned on the railing, and found a way to deal with the news.

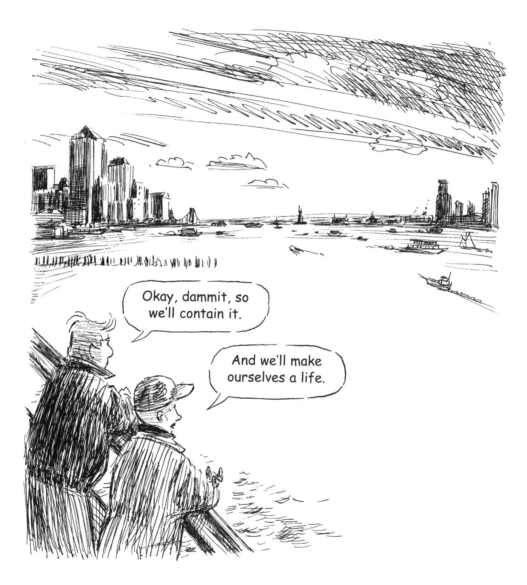

Throughout her treatment, Janet believed she was getting the best medicine available—though she was not naïve about the capabilities of doctors. She also paid attention to the serious and even far-out offerings of friends.

The more I get into this, the more I see the doctors don't have many answers. My doctor doesn't even know whether the Taxol or Herceptin might be making a difference. Then she says, "Oh? You're angry about all this? Well, here're the names of some therapists."

A friend said take $25,000 in cash and go to the Bahamas for a fetal stem cell transfer. But I've done my homework. One day fetal stem cell may fix what kills you, but right now it's not for solid tumors. And bone marrow transplants are like getting hit by a nuclear bomb. I'm also looking into any experimental trials.

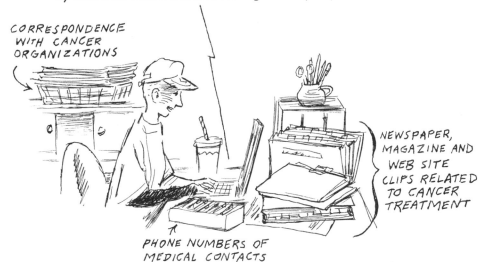

CORRESPONDENCE WITH CANCER ORGANIZATIONS

NEWSPAPER, MAGAZINE AND WEB SITE CLIPS RELATED TO CANCER TREATMENT

PHONE NUMBERS OF MEDICAL CONTACTS

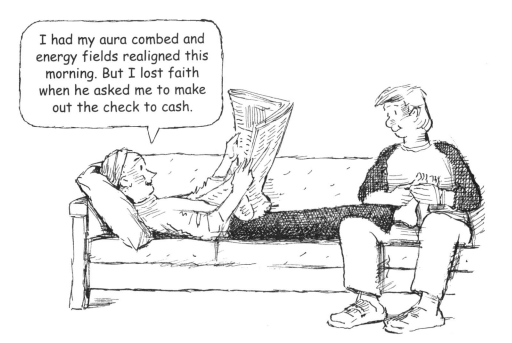

I had my aura combed and energy fields realigned this morning. But I lost faith when he asked me to make out the check to cash.

But the best medicine arrived from an unexpected source. The editor of *Natural History* magazine asked me to do a humorous piece on the solar eclipse that August—during a special eclipse cruise leaving from Greece and sailing the Black Sea. This was the kind of assignment Janet and I dreamed of. My first thought was of Janet. How could I go without her, yet how could she go? Janet took care of that question right away and immediately began the planning that would keep her engaged for the next two months.

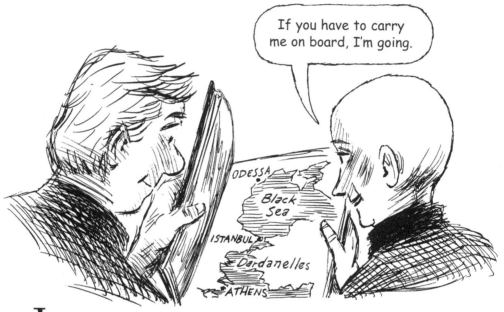

J uly arrived hot and muggy, and we began to understand what Laura meant when she said Janet would never again be normal. Janet's physical deterioration was obvious. She was suffering from increased pain, anemia, sluglike energy, and even gout. We were forced to admit that she could no longer bluff her way through this. The chemo was too destructive. Or something was.

To combat her anemia, we had to start Epogen shots three times a week, which would stimulate red blood cell production. Janet, who was squeamish at the sight of a paper cut, couldn't do it. So I had to. I learned how to fill the syringe, grasp the fat of her arm or thigh, and inject the medicine. She hated those shots, and I hated the hurt I was inflicting. But if she could be brave, so could I.

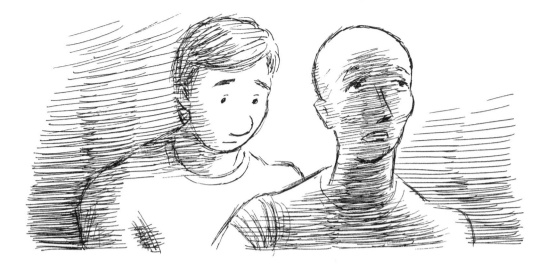

Doctor Stan is giving me the shots. He didn't even practice on oranges first. If I ever go to the great beyond, I'm willing him to my friends . . . In my heart I feel some drug combo will start working. But meanwhile I have to be strong and learn what I'm supposed to learn and not get too angry or sad. And keep looking for the perfect hat.

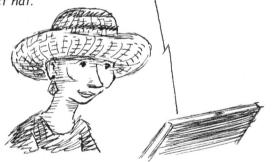

Occasionally someone would make the mistake of asking me for Janet's "prognosis." I'd angrily wave the word away.

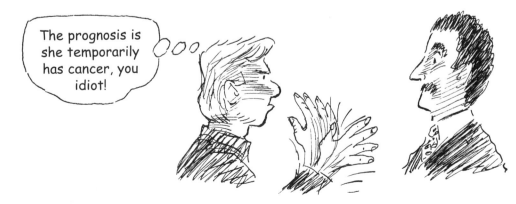

The prognosis is she temporarily has cancer, you idiot!

For me, this was a time to accept my own limitations. I didn't know how to handle this "thing" emotionally, but I could break it down into manageable tasks: shopping for her favorite foods, helping her keep track of meds, fielding phone calls . . . and staying calm.

But I always felt a step behind, unprepared for the next development. As I solved one problem, a worse one took its place.

Janet was having trouble steering our old car, so I traded it for one with power steering. But quickly she was too weak to drive at all.

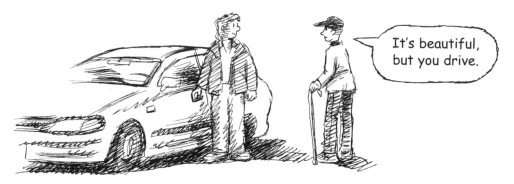

It's beautiful, but you drive.

One day I noticed her paying some bills. Her handwriting was always difficult to read; now it was almost impossible. What if I had to take over her bills? We'd shared every other part of our life, including expenses, but never a bank account.

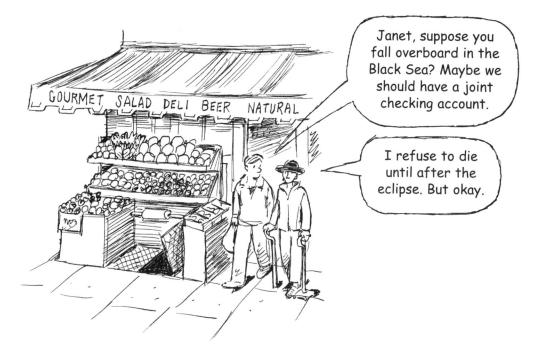

Janet, suppose you fall overboard in the Black Sea? Maybe we should have a joint checking account.

I refuse to die until after the eclipse. But okay.

We walked the four blocks to the bank, and she was winded before we got there. As we sat in the bank officer's cubby, I watched her hand as she filled out the forms. She was giving up pieces of her independence, and it made me so damn sad.

She and I also agreed that I should make an appointment to see Joe, a friend and estate attorney, to talk about how we'd pay for an extended illness. At the same time I'd talk to him about redrafting both our wills—I could never acknowledge that we might need hers before mine—and I'd ask him whether he thought we needed to get married for practical reasons.

"I told Stan that, knowing Janet, I thought it was better for her psychologically to maintain control over her assets. Also, if the paperwork were properly drafted, they wouldn't have to get married for financial reasons. A durable power of attorney would allow him to handle her money while she was alive, and a will would give him the power to handle her financial affairs were she to die."

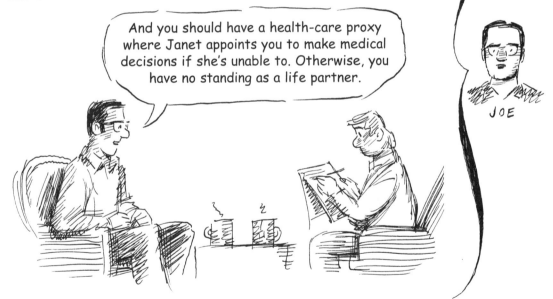

And you should have a health-care proxy where Janet appoints you to make medical decisions if she's unable to. Otherwise, you have no standing as a life partner.

JOE

As Janet and I entered our tenth month in cancerland, Lucy and Carole, Janet's longtime friends, arrived from San Francisco for a visit. Lucy, always the earth mother to Janet and their friends, had recently been the executor for a friend who'd died of AIDS, and she herself had just been diagnosed with multiple sclerosis. She arrived determined to help her dear friend, who she had decided wasn't facing her situation realistically.

"I immediately comered Stan and asked him what he'd done about Janet's money."

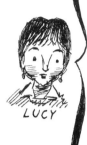

LUCY

You're not married. You have to make sure things get done the way Janet intends. Once people die, it's out of your hands, and something always goes wrong. Relatives can get crazy. Do it immediately.

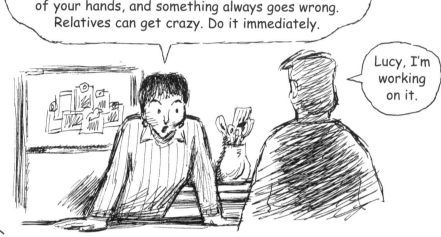

Lucy, I'm working on it.

Even though I understood what Lucy was saying, it was hard to look at the possibility of Janet's death at all, never mind its aftermath. To do that was a betrayal of her. Yet, in time, Lucy's words would return to haunt me.

The three old friends went to Fire Island for the weekend, where Lucy confronted Janet as only Lucy could.

Janet, this may be the last time we're together. Why do we have to wait for you to die to have a party?

Stan doesn't want to talk about dying and neither do I. Wait till the beginning of the year to visit again; things could improve.

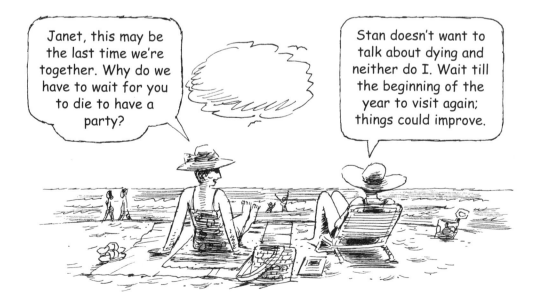

Janet didn't have room in her day for thoughts of dying. She was busy with our plans for the Black Sea voyage on a ship that now included NASA scientists and two former astronauts.

Getting ready for our trip to the Black Sea. Yippee! Sister Carolyn with boyfriend Mike and friend Kathryn with boyfriend Larry have decided to join us. We'll rendezvous in Athens. The New York Times said the region is dangerous for travel right now. I say better to die on an adventure than incrementally by cancer.

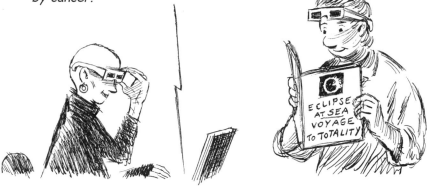

Two weeks before our flight to Greece, Janet came down with a mysterious fever that we couldn't control at home. Laura had her admitted to the hospital. For nine days, they tried every test in the book.

The nurses kept taking blood from her poor veins till she was crying in pain. They refused to use the port because it might be the source of the infection. By day four, I protested that they should have figured that out by now. They insisted it was "doctor's orders." I blew up.

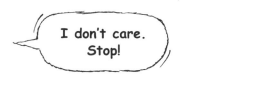

I don't care. Stop!

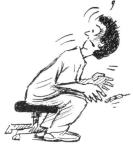

They didn't like it but they stopped, and I realized that patients do have power to make decisions about their own care. I saw how quickly in a hospital setting one becomes a chart rather than a person. But there was one staffer with whom Janet became friendly. Danny was a new intern and Janet was one of the patients assigned to him.

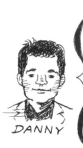

DANNY

"Janet's friendliness was so genuine that she made me feel special. She had a diffuse metastasis to the skeleton and the general sense is that it's rare for the patient to get better. I think she should have been told that her situation was dire. But I also knew that it would be a rare doctor who would do that. It tormented me. I remember when Janet was talking about their Black Sea trip and I thought, What courage . . . and healthy denial."

Meanwhile, we helplessly watched our departure date draw closer.

Every day I caught up on housework and phone calls, then bused to the hospital, bringing her a milkshake or a flower or more itinerary details on our trip. At night we watched *Seinfeld,* and I'd leave around midnight and make my way home. My deep fatigue and the loneliness of the New York streets sliced through my defenses and I felt despair.

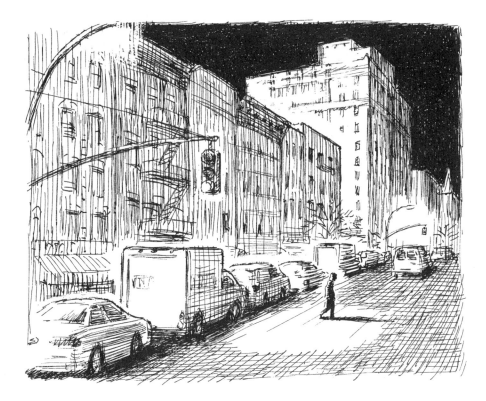

On day ten, the doctors thought they'd found the cause of Janet's infection and fever. They pulled a tooth. Janet consulted with Laura, who knew how important the trip was to Janet.

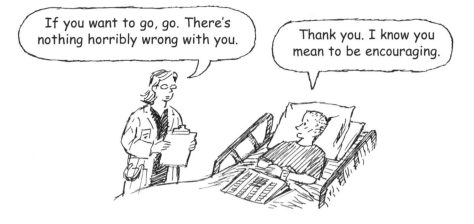

With one day left, we prepared to meet Carolyn and the others who were already there. We gathered our clothes, including her big hat, sunglasses, earrings, lymphedema sleeve, the cooler with her medication and syringes, her many pills, and the name of an oncologist in Athens. Janet excitedly phoned Athens: "Hotel Acropolis House? Yes, a message for Carolyn Bode. Tell her we're coming!"

At the airport, partly for fun, we ordered a wheelchair to take us to the gate. With Janet comfortably seated, the attendant whisked us by a side door past lines of waiting travelers and onto the plane.

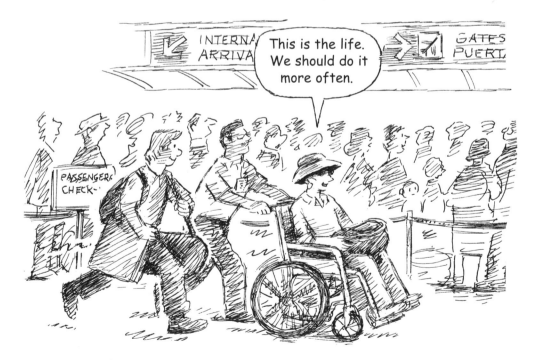

CHAPTER 6

The Elephant in the Room

Janet and I met Carolyn and Mike, Kathryn and Larry in Athens, and we boarded the ship. Cancer or not, Janet and I were embarked on another adventure. We sailed for the Black Sea, stopping at the Temple of Asclepius (the Greek god of healing), the Blue Mosque in Istanbul, the Potemkin Steps in Odessa. Janet, using a cane and moving slowly, came ashore every time.

On the day of the eclipse, while I worked on my assignment, our friends carried Janet in a wheelchair up an outside ladder to the observation deck for a front row seat to the spectacle. She wore a wide-brimmed hat, long scarf, single hoop earring, dark glasses, and black lymphedema sleeve. She looked mysterious and beautiful.

We arrived home on Friday, August 13. In an e-mail a few days later, she described the experience.

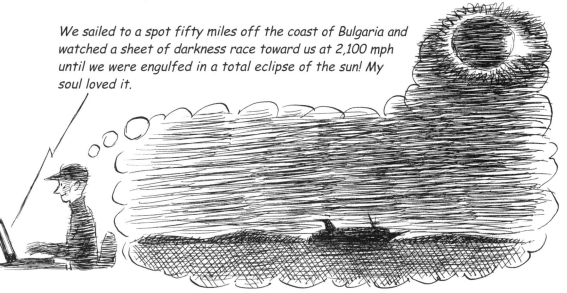

We sailed to a spot fifty miles off the coast of Bulgaria and watched a sheet of darkness race toward us at 2,100 mph until we were engulfed in a total eclipse of the sun! My soul loved it.

But she came home with a raging fever and in hellish pain.

Our friend Linda gave Janet a good-looking wooden cane, and Janet began to depend on it.

I'd do it again in a heartbeat. But I have to accept reality. I can barely walk around the block.

Laura evaluated Janet's condition and told us that the current chemo wasn't working well enough to continue. We now understood that it was the cancer itself, rather than the chemo, that was causing much of her pain.

But Laura told us there were still treatment options. She put Janet on a second chemo drug, Navelbine, and brought in a pain specialist, who recommended methadone. Knowing its addictive properties, Janet called Howie, the ex-heroin addict. They laughed about its street reputation and he assured her that her dosage was very low. Methadone turned out to be far more effective in combating Janet's pain than the morphine she'd been taking. Thinking back, what a sick joke. We were worrying about stuff like addiction when someone should have been preparing us for the last stages of her life.

Laura's discussions with Janet about treatment side effects like nausea, pain, and even about alternative remedies, were straightforward and helpful. And Janet said their conversations were good therapy. However, Laura's approach to the true course of Janet's disease remained ambiguous.

You don't have a curable cancer anymore, but with medication there is a subset of women who . . .

Janet's fate was like the proverbial invisible elephant living in our apartment. Something was crashing around and hurting us both, but we didn't know what. We needed someone to talk honestly, not just about the details of coping with neuropathy, constipation, and bone pain but about the !@#$%! elephant.

How much improvement could we expect from the new chemo? What physiological changes should we prepare for and how should we handle them? Was she terminal and, if so, how much time did she have? Who was to tell us what we didn't know to ask?

One day in September, Janet and I were on the street and she noticed a few early dead leaves on the sidewalk. "Oh dear," she lamented, "fall is here!" We used to joke about how Janet always hated fall. To me, it was a time of brilliant colors and a welcome coolness. To her, it was a gloomy herald of winter's doom. That fall Janet's health would slide inexorably down.

At first, with painkillers, steroids, and blood transfusions, Janet perked up, and she continued with her life—walking, corresponding with friends and colleagues, working hard.

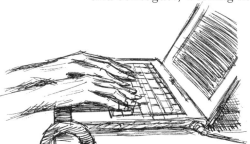

I'm no longer lying in bed composing my obit. I was upright all day, even took the bus to the hospital for tests, and I'm back at my desk.

But gradually Janet's periods of energy got shorter, and she had to acknowledge her limitations.

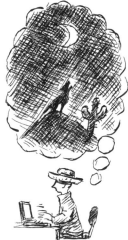

Dixie, thanks for the invitation, I'd love to visit your school in Texas again, but at this moment my wings are clipped. I've learned to make decisions differently when the pain is intense.

Janet, when a bobcat crosses my path on the way home in the dark, or I hear the little pack of coyotes howling and yipping down by the big hill, I think of you and send you hello and my best wishes from the wilds of Texas.

Up till now, Janet was in charge of her illness. I was her chief cook and bottle washer, and faithful backup. Now as pain and treatment wore her down, she needed me to step out in front and take on more of the medical decision making.

She had pills for pain, strength, nausea, bowel movements, spiking pain, tingling of fingers and toes . . . I would wake up in the middle of the night to see her, woozy from drugs, gripping her pen and yellow legal pad, struggling to keep track of the symptoms and medications. And I knew it was only going to get worse.

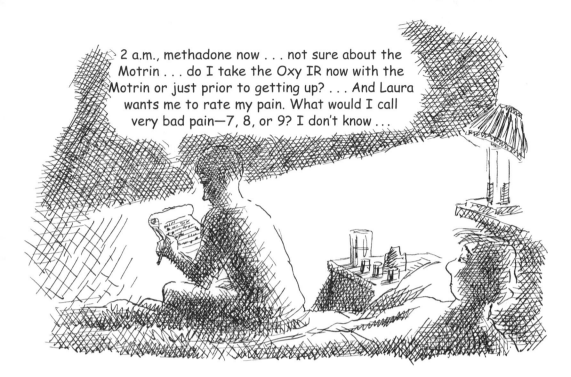

I urged her to get one of those weekly pill organizers. At first she resisted; she'd always relied on her yellow legal pad. Finally she agreed. I took over the job of organizing the pills and made sure she took the right ones at the right time, day and night. It was important to both of us that she was the one to make the decision to delegate the job to me.

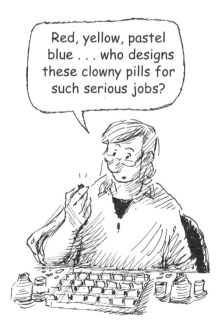

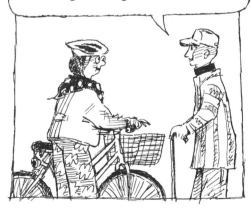

We were now entering a darker world of ever more disheartening medical problems. Janet began to lose bladder control—a situation we tried to make light of.

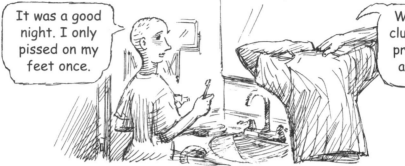

I knew there were handheld plastic urinals that she could keep by the bed at night. I found my way to Bigelow's medical supply store, not far from our apartment. I bought a female urinal and a rubber sheet and came back in triumph. Problem solved.

But the problems never stayed solved. They only got worse.

Janet's nightly incidents increased. I went back to Bigelow's and bought a plastic bedpan. This time I walked the aisles, reading labels on adult diapers, bathroom grab bars, shower seats, walkers, sipping cups . . . giving myself a crash course on what might lie ahead.

Eventually we switched from the bedpan to a full-size bedside commode. I remember walking home on a sunny Saturday afternoon with the commode in my arms, passing strolling couples. I imagined them making cracks to each other about the guy with the toilet.

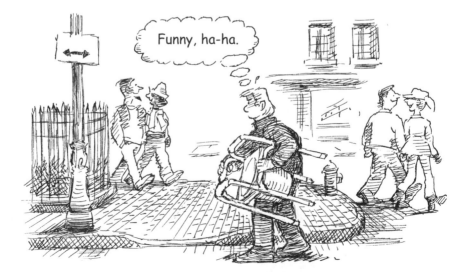

One day, I returned from Bigelow's proud of the good deal I got on a four-footed cane. But soon Janet felt more secure with the extra stability of a walker. Then a wheelchair. Janet joked about doing wheelies, while the canes and walker stood in the corners of the apartment, silent reminders of just last week.

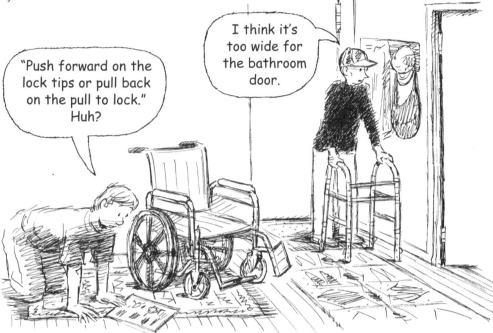

With the wheelchair, the five steps in front of our building, which had been practically invisible to us before, loomed like Everest. I could look for help each time but, practically, we were trapped. I researched city regulations, went online, talked to the building's management. I believed that if I found the right ramp for our sidewalk and door, Janet would be free again.

But it really didn't matter. Once in the wheelchair, she went out less and less.

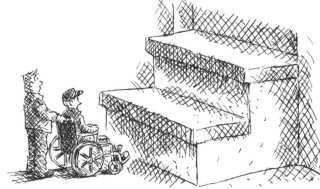

All this time Janet had been going to the hospital for chemo, scans, and blood transfusions. The doctors and technicians cared not at all how we got to them as long as we showed up on time. The cost, the pain, the logistics—all ours. As Janet became less mobile, our transportation changed from bus to cab; once we even hired an ambulance. But we mostly used ambulettes, whose drivers varied from caring to dangerous.

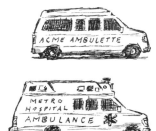

Ambulette: van that transports patients who can sit up. It can securely carry wheelchairs. Driver and helper are not required to have any medical training.

Ambulance: vehicle that transports bed-confined patients by stretcher. Driver and helper are both emergency medical technicians. The vehicle is outfitted with emergency equipment.

Jeannie, a friend from Seattle, came to visit Janet late in October. She went with Janet to one of her blood transfusions. I hadn't had any sleep the night before and needed a nap. Jeannie remembered a harrowing ride home.

"Janet threw up while we waited for the ambulette, which arrived late. The driver was hostile, didn't strap the wheelchair down securely, and had his girlfriend with him. Janet gave him directions, trying to be friendly. Meanwhile, he's a motor mouth and she's bouncing around because of his careless driving.

"Janet realizes he's not taking us straight home, and she has to go to the bathroom. Janet's sleepy with painkillers, and she's fearful of breaking bones. I'm now convinced the driver is on speed.

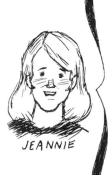

JEANNIE

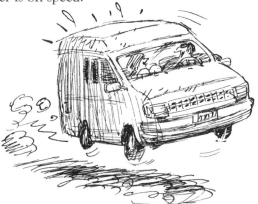

"He finally drops off his girlfriend downtown. Suddenly, Janet wakes up and starts letting him have it. I'm yelling at him too. And *he's* yelling about regulations.

"We make it to the apartment and Janet is swearing about the driver and even grumbling at Stan. I was thinking, Sixty dollars for *that*? This is what it's like being sick in New York?"

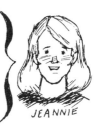

JEANNIE

Even hospitals, supposedly centers of safety and healing, could be hazardous to your health. One day in October, Janet woke up with extreme hip pain. Laura had her admitted to the hospital for observation. In Janet's room, the patient in the adjoining bed was lying in her own waste and appeared to be moaning for help. At the end of visiting hours, they told me I had to leave. I should have insisted on staying, but I left at 11 p.m., planning to be back first thing in the morning. Janet called me in the middle of the night, crying. "I'm on the cuckoo's nest floor. The nurses and attendants are mean, sloppy, and uncaring."

I rushed over early in the morning to find her distraught.

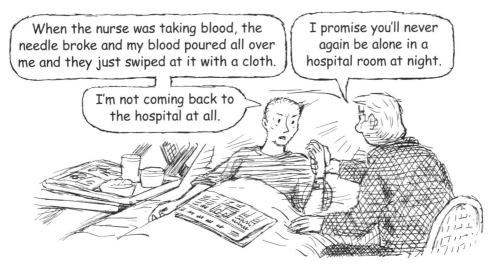

When the nurse was taking blood, the needle broke and my blood poured all over me and they just swiped at it with a cloth.

I promise you'll never again be alone in a hospital room at night.

I'm not coming back to the hospital at all.

In the hospital corridor, I ran into Danny, the intern who'd been on duty when Janet was in the hospital just before the Black Sea trip. I told him I had to get Janet out of there.

Danny used his clout to quickly get Janet released. He said, "This is a high-turnover floor of extremely ill people. It's too busy, a big mess, even dangerous."

Later Laura said, "Oh yes, that's a bad floor, but it was the only bed available."

As we were waiting to leave, I told Danny we really needed help at home. He walked us to a door that said "social worker."

The social worker rushed in, listened to our story, and signed us up with a CHHA (certified home health agency). The social worker said they provide various skilled home services, and she rushed off again—another patient successfully released.

So there actually was a system in place. We just didn't know what it was.

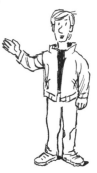

The Way It Works: If the patient requires more nursing help than you can provide, your doctor can authorize home care. The doctor or hospital will contact a CHHA on your behalf. The CHHA will work with your insurance carrier to see how many—or how few—visits your plan covers. The CHHA will assign a visiting nurse to your case. The nurse, in consultation with your doctor, will evaluate your needs and can request such additional services as a visiting physical therapist and home health-care aide and equipment such as a commode and wheelchair.

It looked like we would finally have skilled help—though I didn't even know the difference between a nurse and a home health-care aide.

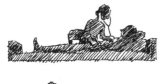

Visiting Nurse: Visiting nurses are directed by the doctor. They evaluate, take vital signs, give medication and injections, and do postsurgery follow-up. Their visits are usually brief.

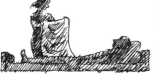

Home Health-Care Aides: Aides do basic health tasks related to the patient such as changing diapers and bedclothes, assisting in feeding and bathing, and doing laundry and errands. They are employed to stay with the patient.

We were contacted by a caseworker, who assigned us a nurse, a social worker, a physical therapist, and a home health-care aide. The nurse visited twice a week. We were one of many on his route; he was almost like a paperboy the way he ran around the neighborhood. He took Janet's vital signs but was not permitted to answer our medical questions.

The social worker arrived and chatted for an hour—mostly about his upcoming retirement.

The physical therapist came weekly. He seemed better suited to working with football players, complained about his own bad back, and left Janet in worse pain.

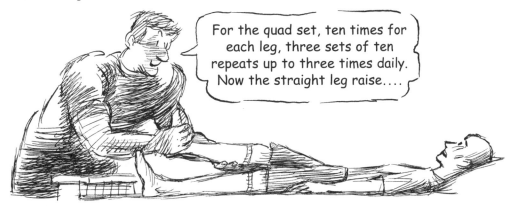

> For the quad set, ten times for each leg, three sets of ten repeats up to three times daily. Now the straight leg raise....

When the home health aide appeared, we were excited—would finally be getting real, practical help. But she was very young, had never worked as an aide before, and didn't seem particularly interested in the job. She began by telling us what she wouldn't do. I fumed, then thanked her for coming and said we wouldn't be needing her services. She refused to leave. Finally our friend Linda took her by the hand and walked her out of the building.

By phone, I was lectured by the agency for not understanding how the system worked. Apparently I did not have the authority to dismiss the aide because all decisions were being made by the CHHA and Janet's insurance company. Though it seems so obvious now, we didn't realize then that we could always go outside "the system," hiring and paying for our own care. Janet and I made decisions based on the information we had.

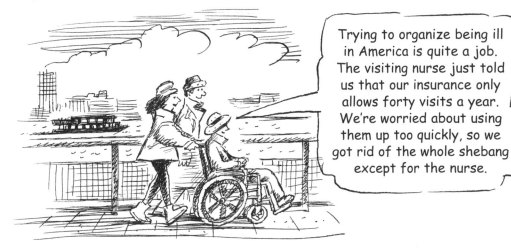

> Trying to organize being ill in America is quite a job. The visiting nurse just told us that our insurance only allows forty visits a year. We're worried about using them up too quickly, so we got rid of the whole shebang except for the nurse.

Janet was eating less, and her tastes were changing. First she craved comfort foods like macaroni and cheese. Then she turned to soups and puddings, and then yogurt, health drinks, and fruit drinks. As she consumed less, I became a Jewish mother.

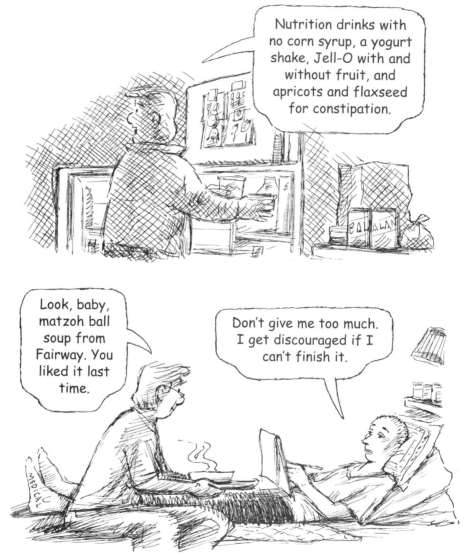

One day in October, a scary thought hit me: maybe she was trying to starve herself to death. I sat on the side of the bed and struggled to come out with the question. She looked at me with genuine surprise and said no. I realized she could never do such a life-denying thing and suddenly I was bawling—something I'd never done before in my life.

She didn't say anything, but the expression on her face made me won-der if she felt she now had to protect me.

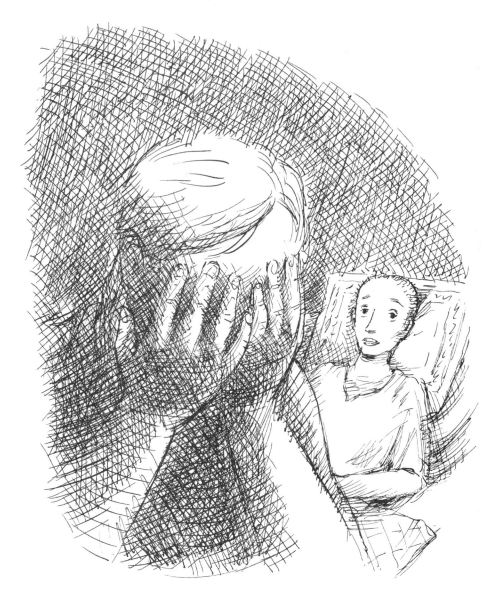

Meanwhile, at the suggestion of an editor, I began work on a new book, a humorous look at the parenting of young children. I could do much of it from the apartment, conducting interviews by phone. Around my daily tasks, I'd squeeze in conversations with mothers of newborns who talked about coping with feeding, diapering, laundry, health worries...

They told me how tired they were, how important schedules are, how constantly vigilant one had to be, how difficult it was for the parents to find time for each other. I understood it all.

And in our bed, Janet lay surrounded by papers, fighting to hold on to her old self and to keep working.

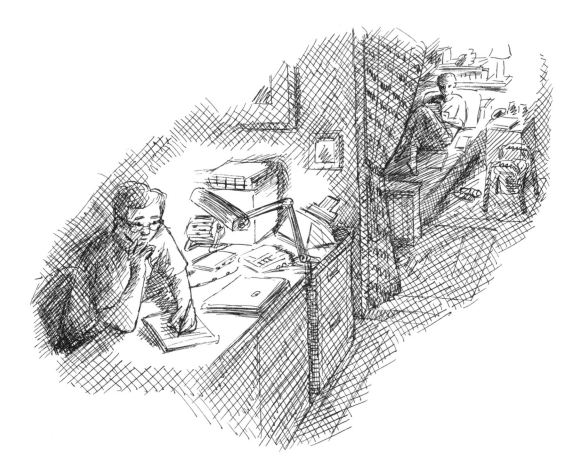

CHAPTER 7

Overtaken

In November, despite increasing difficulty, Janet and I made her weekly chemo and her visits with Laura. And the visiting nurse was still showing up twice a week. But their ministrations didn't make our daily life any easier. Janet was growing weaker and having moments of remoteness. My caregiving and homemaking tasks were draining my strength and occupying all my time. We were beginning to lose touch with each other. I knew we needed help and looked to friends and neighbors—with mixed results.

Some simply could not face Janet's illness.

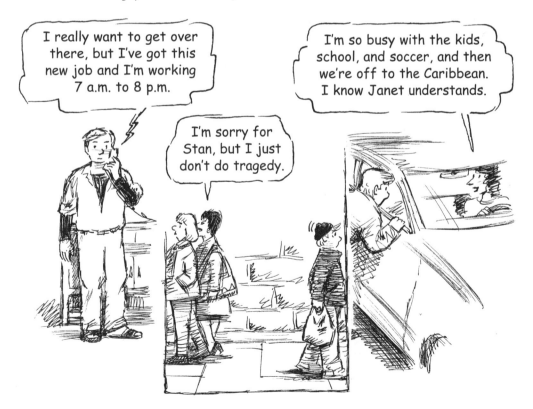

Our good friend Florrie from downstairs said that some of our neighbors acted as if cancer were contagious.

"People in the building would ask me how Janet was. I'd say, 'Ask her.' One said:

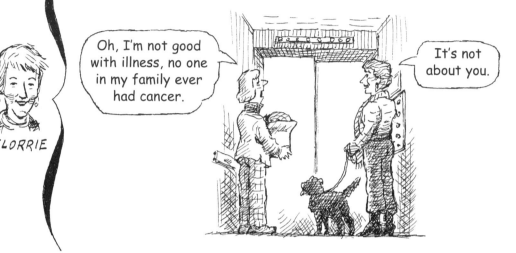

Others meant well but went about it all wrong. One old friend came in from out of town, spent hours in our kitchen making a ham and potato casserole that Janet couldn't eat, and then decided to catch an earlier train.

Then there were the warrior women who gathered around us from different times of her life and different parts of the country. They arrived bearing food and memories, prepared to massage and cook and file and clean and share writers' war stories . . .

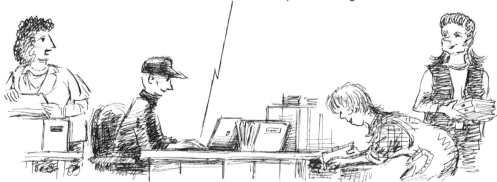

Janet's old friend Linda started coming over almost daily. She pampered Janet and helped me. Linda also thought she knew how things should be done and was quotably blunt about expressing it. But she showed up, and I loved her for it.

"Stan had to know everything that was happening and make all the decisions. He knew every product in every aisle of every market in the neighborhood. And Janet was the same way. She'd give me specific instructions and rules and what she was willing to do. The two of them with their ideas drove me crazy. I remember once muttering to myself:

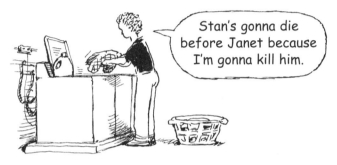

Stan's gonna die before Janet because I'm gonna kill him.

"I'd walk over mornings bringing Janet a daisy or a special drink—something she could keep down. I'd bring Stan a coffee from the corner—good or bad, he didn't know the difference.

"Janet and I spent a lot of time in her bed, watching TV and gossiping about friends. She was often in pain so I'd crawl in carefully around her notebook, books, lotions, drinks . . . I'd do her nails and makeup. After years of nothing but eyeliner, Janet wanted the full course: mascara, powder, rouge, and lipstick. But Janet would not talk about her real condition."

LINDA

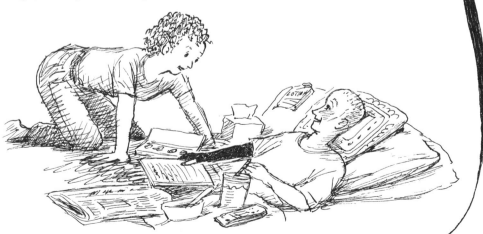

Linda would even get on the phone with the hospital's billing department—in her own inimitable style.

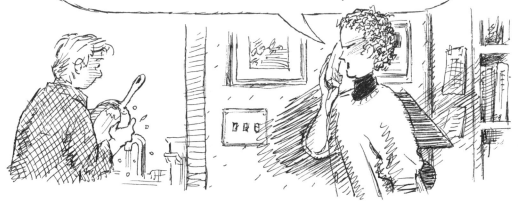

> Janet is very ill and is being hassled by your collection agency. Send the bills to her insurance company. They can't refuse to pay. They're an insurance company! Just make sure they have all the accurate information. I have a bill here where your dates are different from the date of service. **Don't you people know how to run an accounts receivable department?!**

Jane O', a vibrant friend from Janet's writers' group, arrived from her new home in Vermont.

"I came ready to fill the air with the sounds of vacuuming. When I walked in, Janet was in her wheelchair, giving orders to friends. 'Put the towels in there. I need all those letters to kids answered.' I said:

JANE O'

> How is it you're so chipper?

> I'm in denial.

"Then Janet said, 'Come lie down with me. Rub my legs and tell me a story,' which I did. I said to her, 'You're so brave. If it were me, I'd prefer roaring against malevolent forces with furious whining and shouting on the side.' 'I love your language,' said Janet."

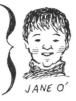

JANE O'

Janet's own words were taking on a new tone. Sitting in her wheelchair, she would e-mail old friends, seeming to want to tie up loose ends.

I wish I'd had the time yesterday to tell you how much our old friendship means to me. I remember that time I left you with all the sorority work during rush week and went off with a date. I disappointed myself for having done that to you.

I still feel I have a long way to go on this journey of mine. I'm just not sure what direction it will take. But with the love, support, and prayers of people, especially you, I feel I can get through it in the most positive way. Thanks for the visit and the chicken salad.

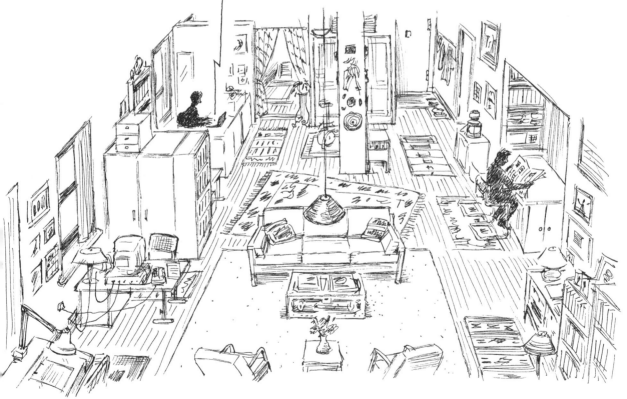

The warrior women continued to help me and form a comforting circle around Janet. But it became clear that friends did not have the time or skill to take the place of professional help. So far, I was still the primary nurse/ home health aide/maid.

Laura once said Janet and I were strong and self-reliant, not like the patients who turned to the hospital for every little thing.

It was true that we were self-reliant, but I was not getting enough sleep, I was losing weight, and I almost never left the apartment.

Everybody was concerned about me.

Some women volunteered to stay with Janet so I could go out, which I did, sort of.

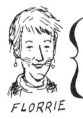

FLORRIE

"I remember when it was my turn to sit with Janet. First Stan took forever to get out the door. And when he finally left, he met a friend for coffee and came right back. Another time he took a walk around the block and was back even faster."

My dear sister, Gloria, would send me care packages from Rhode Island, full of meals I could prepare for myself in our new microwave, itself a gift from another friend. The microwave was a godsend. I'd never cooked much to begin with, and in any case, there was no time. Now I discovered dry soups and frozen dinners.

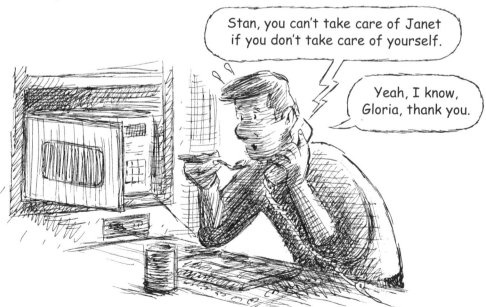

Stan, you can't take care of Janet if you don't take care of yourself.

Yeah, I know, Gloria, thank you.

"You could see that Stan was exhausted. He needed therapy, a mensch to talk to. But we didn't know where his head was. He never let on how he felt. He seemed to be moving along alone without any support. I remember once he and Richard got together."

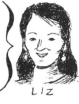

LIZ

"Stan and I met at a diner. When my first wife, Andrea, was dying of cancer, I badly needed my friends. But when I met with Stan, I couldn't pry words out of him with a crowbar. He asked me technical questions about equipment or food. But not, 'I need a drink. What am I going to do?' I don't know where he was putting all that sadness. I wondered, Doesn't he ever scream at the horizon?"

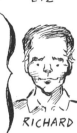

RICHARD

I did scream, but not at the horizon. I yelled at Linda, at telemarketers, at anyone with stupid questions.

Janet had been trying to find out from our insurance company which of our expenses—like the ambulettes—might be reimbursable. Someone from the HMO called the apartment:

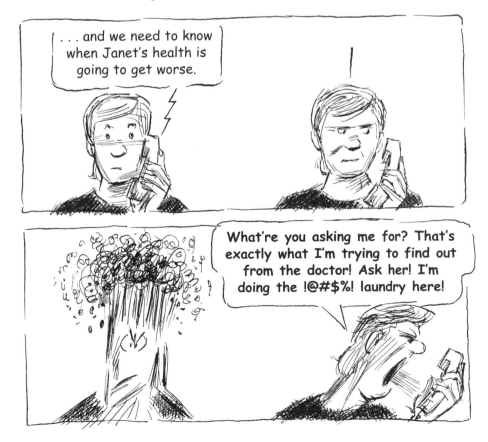

. . . and we need to know when Janet's health is going to get worse.

What're you asking me for? That's exactly what I'm trying to find out from the doctor! Ask her! I'm doing the !@#$%! laundry here!

I was also acting peculiar.

I began to walk the six flights of stairs in our building, up and down, up and down, sweating, making my heart pound, until knee pain forced me to stop.

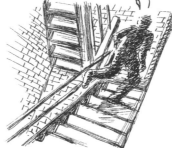

I practiced the Asian martial art of tai chi in the living room with a book of instruction propped up in front of me.

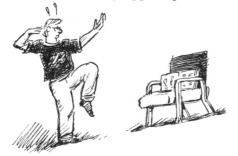

In bed, in the middle of the night, with Janet in a drugged state beside me, I did relaxation exercises from tapes in a boom box on the floor next to me.

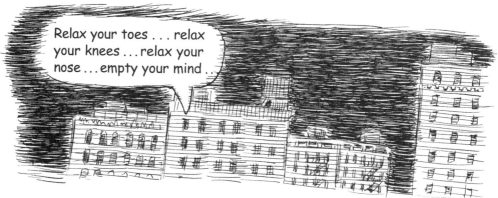

When Carole once more arrived from California, I overheard her say on the phone, "I don't think Stan understands how sick Janet is. But what difference does it make? They're never apart, and they live day by day anyway."

Late in November Kate came for a visit.

"The drugs were beginning to make Janet anxious. When she would become nervous, Stan would say:

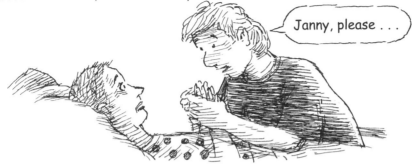

Janny, please . . .

" . . . and she would calm down. She was best when he was near. There was a deliberate openness between them. My sense was she was also taking care of him.

"When I was rubbing her, she said to me: 'It was good with Stan, I love him, I am fortunate to have him. I have friends who care, I am at peace, I've had a good life.'

"Their apartment was a remarkably dignified place. When people arrived, Stan would orient them, bring them up to his level of caring. A visitor once said she's dying, and he got very angry. That was exactly not the point.

"Despite the meditation tapes and the tai chi, I was worried that it was getting too much for Stan. I walked him to the river and said, 'You're getting depleted, you have no network of help. People on drugs can die suddenly and you won't be prepared.' I suggested hospice. He was afraid I was saying that he was supposed to have end-of-life conversations, and he would laugh nervously."

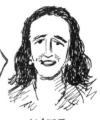

KATE

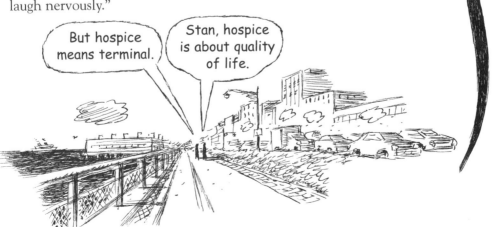

But hospice means terminal.

Stan, hospice is about quality of life.

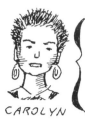

CAROLYN

"In November when Kate was visiting, Janet was severely constipated. Luckily, Kate's a nurse. She manually unblocked her. The visiting nurse was never there when we needed him. I thought, Are we supposed to know how to do everything ourselves?"

Janet's bodily functions had become part of our daily conversation. Janet was still Janet, and she included her friends in the intimate details of her medical life. To her, a good story was a good story, whether it was sailing the Li River in China or the achievement of a successful bowel movement.

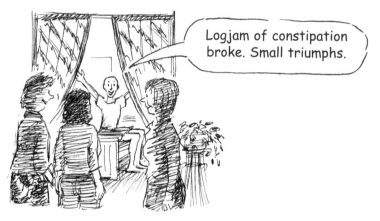

Logjam of constipation broke. Small triumphs.

Even when friends were helping, it was difficult having visitors all the time. Janet would say, "We're tired. I love my dear friends, but Stan and I need to have our private time." The door would finally close on the last visitor, and we'd be alone.

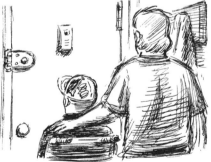

In the quiet of those moments, Janet and I would reach out to each other and try to reconnect, try to feel ordinary again—talking about her twenty-pound weight loss that month and her urine-soaked towel the way we used to discuss publishers' contracts or the occasional mouse in our apartment.

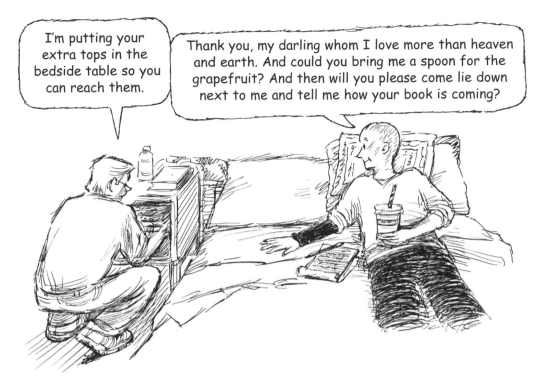

We'd lie in bed watching reruns of *Law & Order* and *ER*—familiar was good. And we talked about the past as though it were the future.

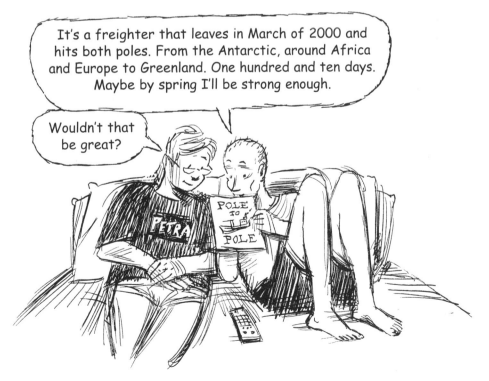

Or we'd talk about nothing.

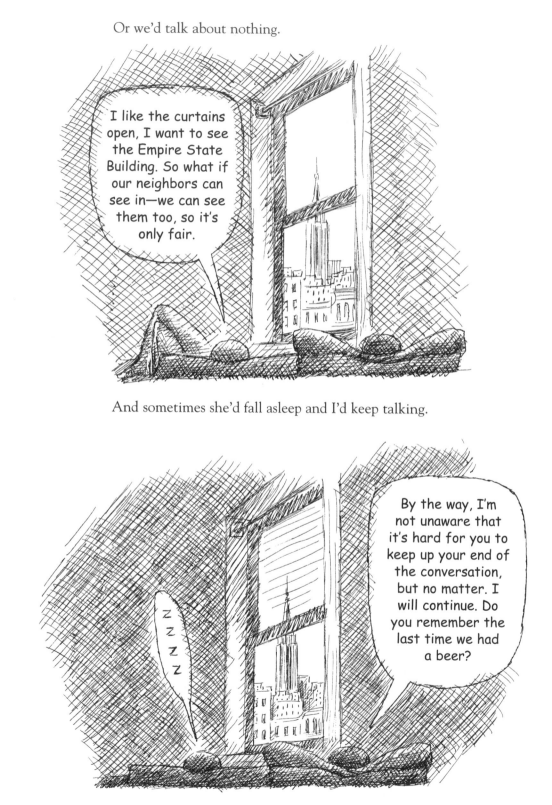

And sometimes she'd fall asleep and I'd keep talking.

Eventually the stress caught up with me and I had a series of anxiety attacks, with a racing heartbeat and a weakness in my arms so bad I couldn't lift anything. It was too much for my little relaxation tapes to handle. Janet was in pain and had missed a few chemo appointments because she was too weak. She and I had gone as far as we could go without help. The elephant had become visible.

Laura had recently told us that we were coming to a time when Janet should have an MRI and an evaluation of the effectiveness of the chemo. We sent her an e-mail telling her that we needed that meeting to understand what was happening and our options.

To our dismay, Laura's assistant left us a message that Laura was away on emergency leave but was getting her e-mails and would call us as soon as she could.

After we didn't hear for a week, we called and sent e-mails.

Laura, left messages but haven't heard from you. Every morning for the past four I've been sick to my stomach. Today was the worst. Threw up four times from 4 a.m. to 12 p.m. I'd like to talk to you about stopping the Navelbine for a while. Maybe it's time to start another drug. I'm losing too much weight. If you're not available to meet, at least let's talk by phone.

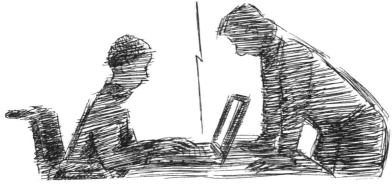

No response.

"Stan kept me informed about what was going on. Janet had looked to Laura as a friend as well as a doctor. Now they couldn't reach her and it was awful. As a nurse I sometimes feel like saying, 'I know I'm giving you shitty care but don't ask me anymore, I've given all I can.' And I know Laura had her own problems. But Janet was the most forgiving of souls and Laura was hurting her. You couldn't defend that."

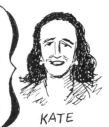

KATE

105

Janet and I were becoming desperate over not being able to get in touch with Laura. On November 21, I sent an e-mail, hoping to get her attention, or at least that of her assistant:

> Laura, Based on Janet's current condition, I think it's time to ask you some serious questions. This past week Janet had bad pain. Increased sleepiness. Morning vomiting. Generally weaker and more bedridden. Needs more constant attention. So my questions are: Are we going on with chemo, and if so, is it worth it? Since she now needs more home care than I can do myself, should you put me back in touch with a social worker? I don't know my options. Under what circumstances do we start to think about hospice care? What might be the meaning of her not eating—her diet has been more and more sliced fruit, apple-sauce, Jell-O, juices, milk, and sodas. Will her body waste away? And while I know you can't be sure, what are the probabilities of her situation? What does all this mean for the near and far future? You should know that I suffered from a series of anxi-ety attacks this week. It scared me. Talk about these issues would help all of us. Janet also approved this note. Stan

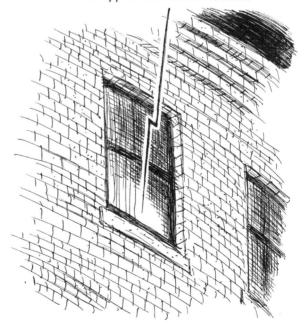

We received an e-mail from Laura saying she was back in her office and that we should have a short admission for Janet to assess everything, or if the transport was too painful that I should come in and discuss it—that it deserved an in-person discussion.

I said I was ready to meet her any time.

Then, two e-mails: one from her assistant saying Laura was away on leave again; another from Laura telling us that a doctor we barely knew was covering for her, but that she, herself, would set up a time for us to talk ASAP. But it never happened.

We didn't want to see some other doctor—this wasn't an isolated medical question, this was a life issue that only the doctor who'd been with her the whole time could address. I sent another e-mail a week later—and got back only silence.

I'm sorry for your problems but hope you have some time for us. Janet's concerned, I'm frightened. My sense is that her condition is somehow changing. She's more passive, sleeping, lying quietly, taking only fluids. From time to time she's her old self, but still with confusion and an inability to concentrate. If you think she must go into the hospital for tests, she wants to go onto the good floor. And I want her to have a private duty nurse. Even with her friends helping, I'm a little overwhelmed.

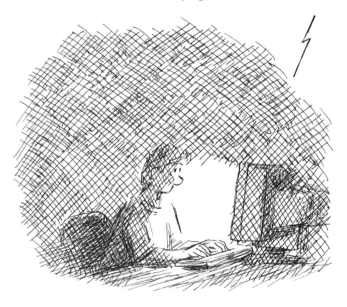

CHAPTER 8

The Angels Come Calling

The silence continued for another week. We'd become desperate. Finally I called Janet's surgeon, Beverly, and told her we couldn't reach Laura. She said she'd find her. On the second of December, our phone rang. I answered it and it was Laura. She apologized for being out of touch and said that she was still on emergency leave. During the call, Janet was sitting across the room in her wheelchair. She was facing away from me and toward the window.

Then Laura said:

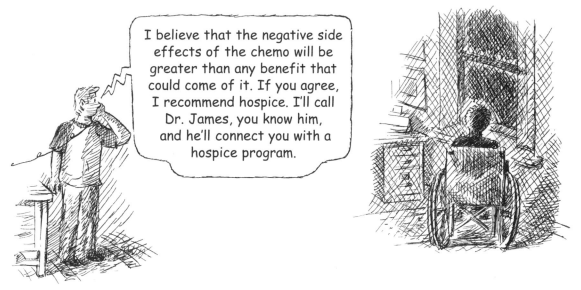

I believe that the negative side effects of the chemo will be greater than any benefit that could come of it. If you agree, I recommend hospice. I'll call Dr. James, you know him, and he'll connect you with a hospice program.

I said yes, and that's the last time we heard from Laura. Though I couldn't see Janet's face, I knew that she understood what had been said.

For years, we had believed she could be cured. For the past months, we believed she could have a life, even if with limitations. I now chose to believe, or, at least my heart chose to believe, that, with luck, we could still keep death at arm's length. Maybe miracles are no more than tiny resistances collected like the grains of sand on all the beaches of the world.

I hung up the phone and said to Janet, "Not having the chemo will give you time to rest and build up your strength. Then we'll see." She nodded.

That night Janet called Rosemarie and said, "I'm not good, Roe. I'm gonna die, I know it. I don't like it, but those are the facts. Nothing else can be done. This is it."

By the next morning, Janet had found something to live for, the publication of her new book on teens and the immigrant experience. From the bed Janet said to me, "Don't worry, swee'pea, I'm fine, just a little tired. Would you please hand me the phone?" She called her friend Jeannie in Seattle.

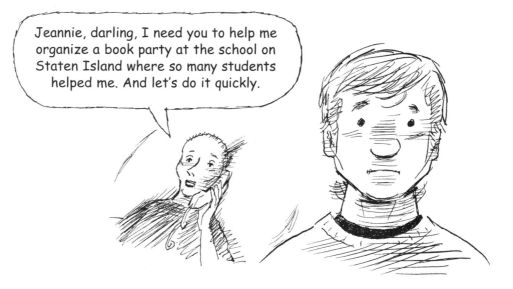

Jeannie, darling, I need you to help me organize a book party at the school on Staten Island where so many students helped me. And let's do it quickly.

That afternoon, Linda and I went to see Dr. James, who simply repeated what Laura had said. He had his assistant contact Jacob Perlow Hospice. He told us the hospice people would be in touch. All I knew about hospice was that they offered care to people who were dying and that Kate recommended them. I was to find out that, in order to be eligible for hospice care, the doctor has to say that the patient has six months or less to live.

Within a few hours we received a call from the hospice coordinator who said they would send over an admissions nurse.

Two days later, Alice, the Jacob Perlow Hospice admissions nurse, stood in our living room. Lucy and Carole had just arrived from California and were there, too.

"Janet wanted to participate in our discussion so we sat around her bed—I sat on the commode. Everyone was worried but open. I made an assessment of the patient and explained about hospice.

"I don't tell the patient he or she is dying, but I do open the door to talking about it. Doctors' refusal to accept death is maddening. I felt Stan and her friends were scared but willing to talk. Janet was the least scared."

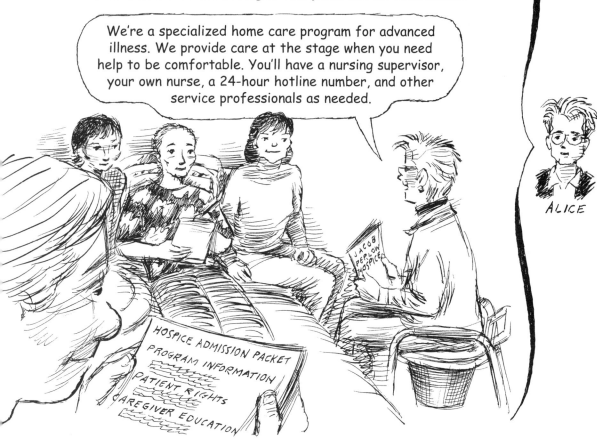

We're a specialized home care program for advanced illness. We provide care at the stage when you need help to be comfortable. You'll have a nursing supervisor, your own nurse, a 24-hour hotline number, and other service professionals as needed.

ALICE

HOSPICE ADMISSION PACKET
PROGRAM INFORMATION
PATIENT RIGHTS
CAREGIVER EDUCATION

Alice spoke with us for two hours, and I felt the weight of desperation begin to lift. She said hospice would arrange things with our health insurance carrier and supply medications. I thought, No more fighting with billing, no more last-minute drugstore runs, no more confusion about dosage adjustments and equipment . . . thank you, thank you.

Once hospice was in place, we no longer had to deal with the home health agency. Instead we were in the embrace of the nurses whom I began to call the angels. Jill was the nurse supervisor. She was the soothing voice on the phone, a friend and advisor we never met. Jane was our nurse. She looked like the glamorous star of a '40s Hollywood movie and arrived by bicycle. She was a virtuoso of a nurse and she and Janet were kindred spirits.

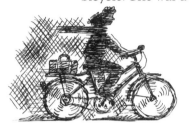

"When I arrived, Janet said, 'Come sit by me.' We sat and I rubbed her and we talked. I found myself telling her about my life and how nursing had saved me during a low time. I had entered at the eleventh hour of Janet's life, yet I felt I'd found a mentor.

"Every time I'd walk in, this loving man and this harem of floating goddesses were showing me the art of caring. Janet went in and out of clarity, reminiscing with her friends, secure because all of them had parts of her memory.

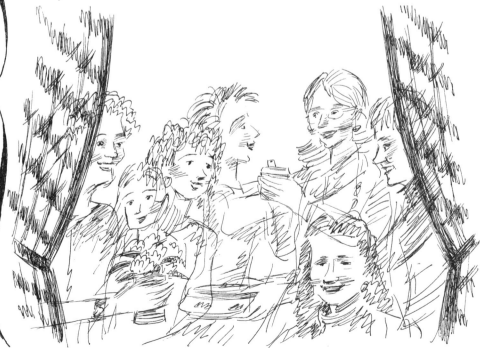

JANE

"My visits after that were about working with everyday problems: adjusting medications, checking for infections, monitoring her constipation—which is a very dangerous condition. She got excited about things she could do for herself, like wiping her mouth with sponge swabs.

"I went over with Stan what was going on with Janet's body, why he should expect changes to speed up, and what he should be doing. He was persevering but exhausted trying to stabilize everything.

"He was always experimenting—Janet had a million kinds of spill-proof glasses. He had the refrigerator filled with juice, Jell-O, applesauce, nutrition drinks, yogurt, and ice cream shakes. Meanwhile, he was eating whatever was around—fat, sugar, decaf coffee, ramen soups. And doing tai chi from a book.

"Stan didn't realize that he was becoming death's midwife."

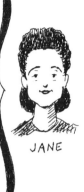

JANE

I was aware that people said I was doing an admirable job caring for Janet (some might say obsessive), and I agreed. But it was also true that I'd begun to sneak glances at my future. I didn't talk about it, but I knew it was coming. I was going to be alone and free—no attachments, no responsibilities. Dream scenarios buoyed me and embarrassed me. They tended to be romantic fantasies. I'd be a foreign correspondent/cartoonist wandering the world, a world-weary yet wise expatriate in some exotic locale, a companion to wealthy women traveling from one luxurious watering hole to another. Then I'd grow discouraged. I was too old to start a new life. I'd come back to earth, shove aside such unworthy thoughts, and return to my real life and love.

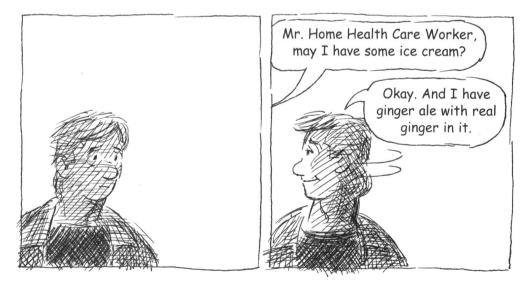

Mr. Home Health Care Worker, may I have some ice cream?

Okay. And I have ginger ale with real ginger in it.

Janet's moments of clarity alternated with times of disorientation, but she never lost sight of her book party. Jeannie had done her job and the event was set for December 12. A few days before the event, Jeannie flew to New York. Carolyn and Kate also arrived to take part. Janet had used her periods of lucidity to write a speech that Carolyn would read.

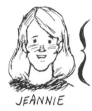

JEANNIE

"When I got to the apartment, Janet said to me, 'I'm not great, but I'm not dying.' I called my husband Bill and said, 'She's dying, but that's not what's happening in their apartment.'"

The morning of December 12, Linda did Janet's hair and makeup, and I helped her on with her favorite purple top—all dressed up for the event she couldn't attend. "Show time," she said. This was her big moment. Jeannie, Carolyn, and a few other women friends gathered at our apartment and then left for Staten Island. Kate stayed back with us. The apartment grew quiet, but Janet was excited.

Late in the afternoon everyone swept back in. Thinking the excitement might be too much for Janet, Kate and I tried to contain their exuberance. But Janet was fully alert and wanted to hear all the details. Her friends draped themselves around the bed and put on the video they'd made. The students talked eloquently about the woman who'd given them a voice in a book. Janet was delighted and teary. She asked for Coke and lemon, her favorite drink from years ago. For that day she was herself, in command, a professional writer doing what she did so well.

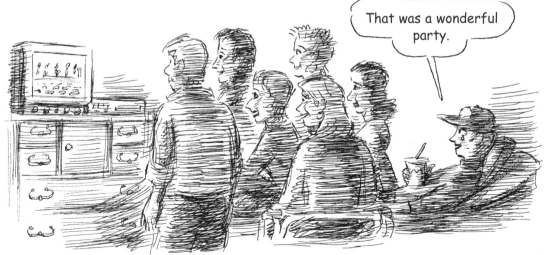

That was a wonderful party.

"On Monday, as I was heading home, I called and Janet immediately got on the line. She gave me advice for getting to the airport and said, 'Thanks for everything, I'll see you the next time around. I love you.' There was nothing to be gained by talking further. My sense was that she wasn't going to give the disease the satisfaction of knowing that she knew it was killing her."

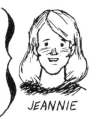

JEANNIE

That Sunday was a triumph for Janet. Monday night, in bed, Janet was still savoring the details and making plans:

> I'm going to call Jeannie. We have to plan another party at the school in Texas that also helped me.

> Okay, sweetheart, but give yourself a day of rest first.

The bed Janet and I slept in was a symbol of normalcy, and I had refused to give it up. To protect Janet's skin, Jane brought in an egg-crate foam mattress that sat on top of the futon, which meant I was left to sleep in an eighteen-inch space between the foam mattress and the edge of the bed. I had to turn over like a piece of lamb on a spit, but that was okay because I could still reach over and squeeze her hand and she could squeeze mine back.

Normalcy was something she and I needed to believe in. She said to Jane, "Stan and I are down to oral sex." I smiled because by then our sex life had tapered off to gentle stroking.

Sometimes, in the middle of the night, lying next to her, I struggled with physical longings, which quickly mingled with exhaustion and feelings of guilt. But Janet understood.

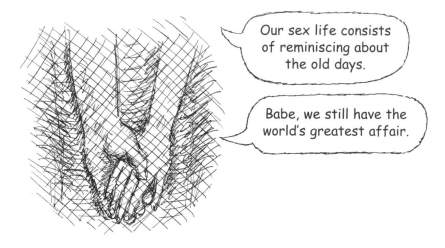

Our sex life consists of reminiscing about the old days.

Babe, we still have the world's greatest affair.

Finally, to protect Janet and make it easier for everyone caring for her, I had to give in to a hospital bed. When it first arrived, I felt sick. The bars of the bed now separated us. The futon bed became another couch in the living room. And the egg-crate mattress became my bed on the living room floor.

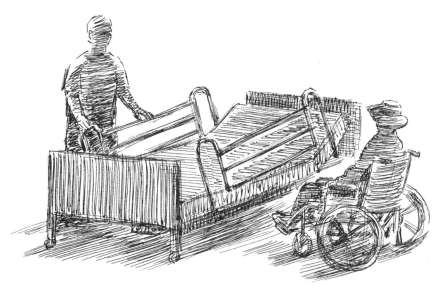

Now I did something I should have done a month earlier—I hired two home health-care aides. I needed round-the-clock help from professionals who knew how to change the sheets with Janet still in bed. Who had the experience to be prepared for Janet suddenly struggling out of bed, and to be able to gently guide her back.

After some trial and error, I decided that this was too important to let the medical insurance people dictate who and for how long. With Jill's help I found two home health-care aides whom I hired myself. By day, Nichole—bustling, outgoing, sunny. And by night, Auda—cool, competent, able to sit silently and alert by the bed for hours.

"The family and friends of the patient usually leave at night. They come in in the morning and say, 'How is she?' Stan was there all the time. He slept behind the couch and jumped up every two hours like he had some kind of internal clock. He never said, 'Why is she doing this to me?'

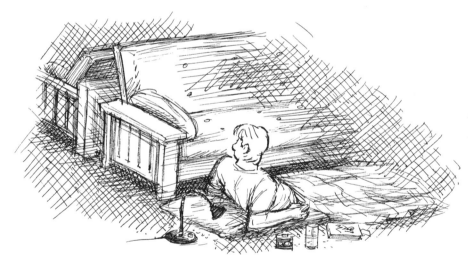

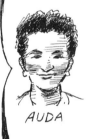

AUDA

"Janet was part of the life of the apartment—as though she didn't think she was dying that soon. I've had other patients who, at that stage, say, 'What's the use?' One patient asked me to kill her with a plastic bag. But we were planning a New Year's celebration, with champagne. Janet and Stan, Carolyn and Mike, Jane, Nichole and me."

The apartment wasn't normal anymore, but it was transformed by the people around us.

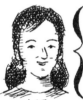

CAROLYN

"I remember walking into Janet's room in December. The light of the window came through colorful scarves from China and Thailand. On her bed was an aqua throw that friends had brought from India, and the intricate quilt a friend had made. There was art from their trips to Australia and Tobago on the walls. Women were lounging around the bed, giggling like sorority sisters, and bringing food and drink. Everyone had an arm or a leg. Janet was drifting in and out. Once when we were chatting over her head, Janet interrupted and said:

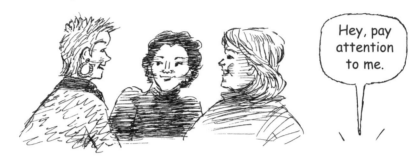

Hey, pay attention to me.

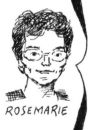

LIZ

"There was a sense of reverie, and a certain joyousness. Women on a mission, pitching in, mothering, no sense of modesty. Someone was always stroking, Janet purring. Visitors brought different kinds of creams until Janet smelled like sweet flowers."

ROSEMARIE

"Someone had sent too many boxes of pudding mix and Stan was trying to find storage space. Janet was still giving directions. 'Roe, come sit with me.' I'm not what you'd call touchy-feely so I said, 'I'm doing the laundry.' Then I felt guilty because I didn't want her to think I didn't love her, so I said, 'Janet, let me comb your hair.' Without chemo, her hair had been growing back.

"She sat in the wheelchair and I brushed her in front of the mirror. It reminded me of when I was a teenager brushing my mom's hair. I thought, I should be asking Janet if she has anything she wants to say to me. But I didn't."

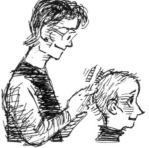

Janet and I had arrived at a plateau—a level and orderly place closer to the clouds. There we focused on the everyday and dwelled together in a kind of peace. She transmitted her strength and calm to me. I don't know where else I would have found it.

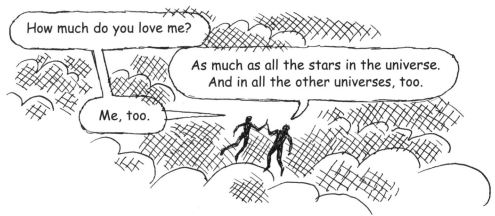

There were moments when she'd look backward and forward with a rueful humor and clarity.

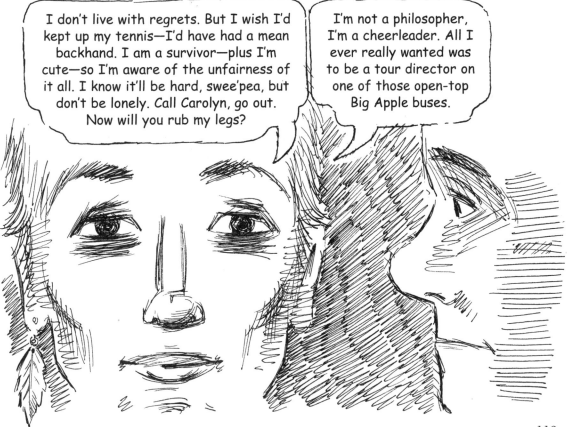

It was becoming increasingly difficult for Janet to swallow pills. I made a ritual out of the pill taking. I cut the pills with my handy-dandy pill cutter, crush some in a little applesauce and drop others into small amounts of juice in tiny paper cups. I rotated juice flavors so she could have her choice. Auda would sit next to me as I made soothing and encouraging sounds to get Janet to swallow a pill. Auda and I celebrated each time a pill went down. Such were our successful days.

JANE

"As we approached Christmas, Janet was having increased periods of distress and lethargy, her color was ashen gray. But she always responded to gentle care and having Stan near. She'd be holding court, then get agitated. And only Stan's touch would bring her anxiety down.

"I said, 'Stan, life and death are a loop. Janet's body is dissolving, going through metabolic changes, preparing to die. It's the end-stage process. You must prepare yourself.' He seemed to understand and was more relaxed."

I allowed that she was dying, but I set the time at a few months away. Still, it wouldn't hurt to prepare. I went to one funeral parlor, but it smelled musty. Linda found a nice, family-run place in Little Italy. One day she walked me there to sign papers. I was on automatic pilot.

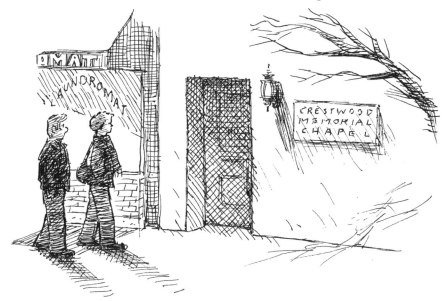

And I talked to Janet's old friend, Betty, a journalist, who began writing an obituary.

Jane O' visited for the last time on December 23:

"It was sunny that day, and it seemed very important to Stan that we sit Janet in her wheelchair in the sunlight. It felt like months had passed since my last visit. She was thinner, kept falling asleep, and couldn't keep anything down. 'Oh, I peed,' she said—less and less caring.

"Janet said to Stan, 'I want some more pills, please, Stan.' And he said:

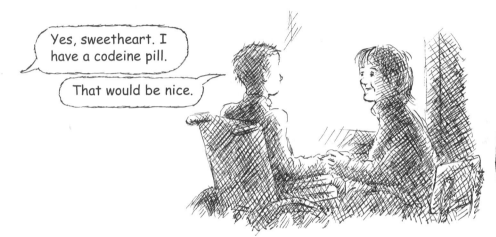

> Yes, sweetheart. I have a codeine pill.

> That would be nice.

"It had gotten dark and she'd been sleeping. She woke up and said, 'Who's out there? I'm afraid.' I asked her if we should have a talk about resignation. I thought she'd spent a little too much time fighting the cancer.

"She said, 'I don't want to die. I'm not afraid of dying, but I don't want it to hurt. I don't know how to die.'

"I said, 'You're the bravest. If anyone can do it, you can. You're going straight to heaven. The gates are wide open. Send us back word. You've done huge things for children and did a lot for me. I love you very much.'

"She said, 'I love you, too.'

"Then she perked up and said:

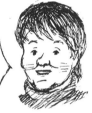

JANE O'

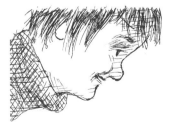

> Hello, dear. I'm not at my best. We're getting a Christmas tree and decorating it.

"When I left I went to a Christmas concert. I wanted to tell people, 'My friend's dying.' I prayed fiercely for an early release. I'd learned to pray in AA."

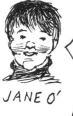

JANE O'

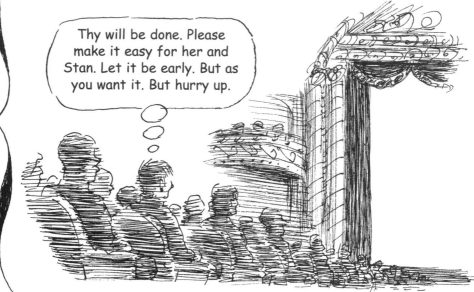

Thy will be done. Please make it easy for her and Stan. Let it be early. But as you want it. But hurry up.

Carolyn's boyfriend, Mike, arrived in New York on December 23 and showed up with a fat, five-foot tree for the living room. Then he went in to say hello to Janet.

"When I walked into the room Janet came awake. She said, 'Thank God you're here. I'm worried.' She thought people were threatening to do things to her—she was mixing TV with reality. She was worried for Stan and Carolyn. I said, 'Don't worry, I'm here to take care of the trouble. You take care of everything else.' She asked me if she was going to die. I didn't know what to say. I said:

MIKE

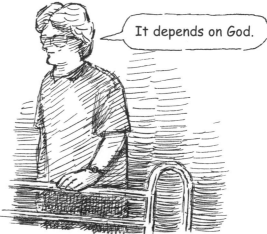

It depends on God.

122

Carole and Lucy flew in and visited on the twenty-fourth. Janet had a burst of energy and determination that carried her through the next two days.

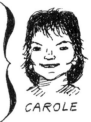

CAROLE

"When we arrived, Janet was sitting up in bed, wearing the red winter jacket we'd sent her. 'Where were you?' she said. My dear friend was dying and she was still giving me shit. She said, 'I want to be like a sandwich between my two best girlfriends.' Then she told us where the Christmas tree ornaments were and we decorated the tree. When we left, I said to Janet, 'Be there on my shoulder.' She said, 'Okay.'"

Early Christmas morning, Janet said she wanted to put on makeup and go out into the living room. Auda washed her hair, put on her pink socks and pink eyeshadow. Janet had on blue fingernail and toenail polish and a bright T-shirt. "Gotta be hip," she said.

Carolyn, Mike, Nichole, and I were in the apartment that day. Carolyn pushed Janet in her chair around the apartment, and we played old Christmas songs. Then Janet grew weak, and we exchanged gifts around the bed. It was difficult for me. Some of my favorite times with Janet were holidays when her enthusiasm would just bubble over. So, even though she was smiling and happy to have us around her, I had to run my wrists under the cold water a number of times that day.

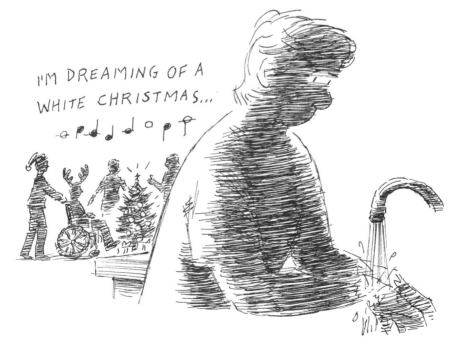

I'M DREAMING OF A WHITE CHRISTMAS...

My son Peter visited Janet on Christmas evening.

"I told her I was going to the Canary Islands over New Year's. She said, 'You'll have a great time.' Then she said:

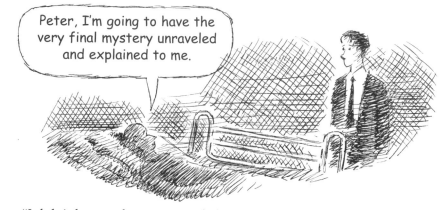

Peter, I'm going to have the very final mystery unraveled and explained to me.

PETER

"I didn't know what to say and changed the subject. 'I'll bring you back some lace, they're famous for their lace.'"

The next afternoon, the Christmas tree lights were blinking on and off in the living room, and Janet and I were alone in the bedroom. I leaned over the rail and told her that a magazine was running an article about how important her books were to teenagers. She opened her eyes and I read it to her. My voice was unsteady, but Janet glowed. I was sure she was thinking, *It's about time.*

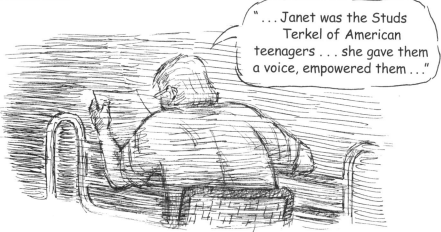

"... Janet was the Studs Terkel of American teenagers ... she gave them a voice, empowered them ..."

What Janet didn't know was that I was reading from the obituary that Betty had prepared.

124

I sat watching her tired face, and remembered a song Carole had written years ago when Janet left San Francisco.

> *Save your tears, I don't want them,*
> *I don't need them anymore . . .*
> *I am moving to a new life,*
> *like I never knew before.*

The lyrics now took on new meaning. I thought, *Maybe it's dawned on her that to die is to go on a great adventure.* I imagined her going through the death-preparation equivalent of making reservations and packing. Actually I was the one who wanted to believe it. I could also imagine her snorting at the very idea.

I thought of Janet's religious grandmother from Sheboygan and decided to cover Janet's bases for her. I called Jill and asked her to please send over the hospice minister. That afternoon, Steven arrived. We talked for a bit in the living room and then he started to walk into the bedroom. It hit me that if he leaned over Janet and started praying, he could scare the bejesus out of her. So I said to him:

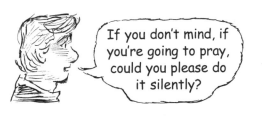

If you don't mind, if you're going to pray, could you please do it silently?

He went in, patted her hand, and sat quietly.

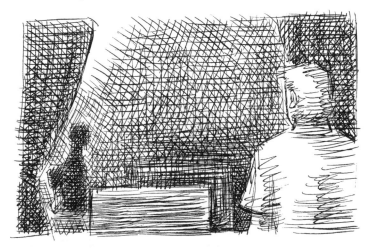

Janet was more and more receding into a mist. When talking was too difficult, she and I used little repetitive phrases to show we were still there. She'd hiccup when she took some meds and then say "Burp." And I'd say "Burp" back, and we'd smile. I'd say "Oy" while rearranging her pillows and she'd repeat "Oy." Or I'd whisper "I love you" in her ear and, even if she appeared to be asleep, she'd whisper back, "I love you, too"—never once missed. And if I cried, as I often did, she'd make small consoling sounds and say, "My precious angel." We were still partners.

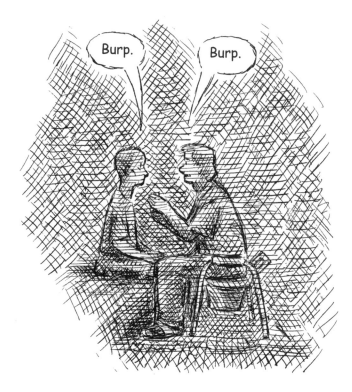

Janet's system was shutting down. Her liver wasn't functioning; the cancer may have reached her brain. She'd ask for juice, but her hand would jump, making it impossible to hold the cup. We'd have to help her find her mouth. Jane said the twitching was called flapping.

Sometimes she would drink from a cup that wasn't there. That was the hardest for me to watch.

I had stopped working on my parenting book. The only thing I was doing was a small monthly comic strip for *The New York Times*—and that only because I could do most of it at night. All that fall I'd talked over my cartoon ideas with Janet and it had the familiarity of our old life. My December strip was due on the twenty-ninth, but I was so tired and distracted I knew I couldn't deliver.

But I was also angry—at the fates for having dealt Janet such an unfair hand and at the outside world for seeming not to care. At night I stared out at the many other lighted windows and wondered which ones contained people suffering and isolated, while the rest of the world planned their New Year's Eve parties.

I decided to do a comic strip about the way it really was for us that would wake people up. I would portray a few typical minutes in our day— the sad, the stupid, the sweet. That would do it.

I sat by the bed and told Janet my idea. She immediately reached for her pad and pen—to participate, as always.

I could hardly believe it—she was sitting up and writing. She wrote for a couple of minutes, looking like her old self, and then began to doze. I took the pad from her hand and saw that she had written many lines of looping *o*'s. There were no words, but I knew what she meant.

For the next two nights, as Janet slept and Auda sat guard, I drew. Jane was there as I was finishing. I asked if she thought I should include the word *mushy*. She said:

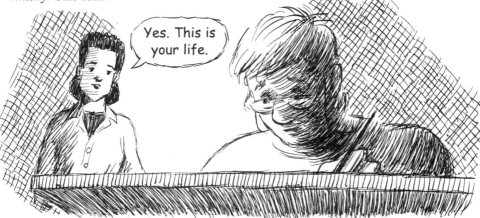

I delivered the strip on Tuesday. It would appear the next Sunday— January 2, 2000.

CHAPTER 9

Dancing in the Dark

In the last days, the atmosphere of our apartment changed. The light, the sound, the movement all became dim. Carolyn was staying in a neighbor's apartment down the hall. Jane, Nichole, and Auda were around us. Janet was quiet, sedated, calm. Life for us was small murmured words, monitored bodily functions, and sips of fruit juice and medications.

My habit was to help Janet out of bed and onto the commode, and while there give her her meds. Now even those two small steps and turn were becoming too difficult. This night would be the last for the commode. Tomorrow, she'd stay safely in bed and we'd use only diapers—one more transition.

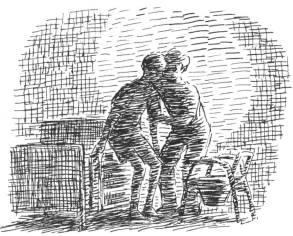

On the night of the twenty-eighth, as always, I woke Janet at 2 a.m. and attempted to guide her to the commode. I got her on her feet, but she was very disoriented and weak. I was afraid she'd fall. I had to do something to get her attention.

I whispered to her, "Janet, sweetheart, dance with me." I took her in my arms . . . and she raised hers to me. I gently lifted her onto my feet and guided her through a slow two-step and turn. Our bodies touched in a way they hadn't in a long time and the embrace felt wonderful.

For that moment the room fell away, and we were again a healthy, happy couple, dancing in the dark.

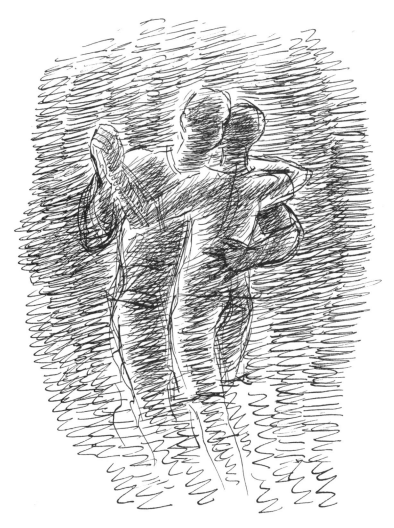

Janet had a small smile, Auda a big one. When Janet was positioned right, I lowered her perfectly onto the commode. I imagine Janet smiled because the only thing we never did well together was dance, till that night.

Janet didn't speculate about death with me, didn't philosophize about life. But the next day she came out of a fog, looked up at me, and said,

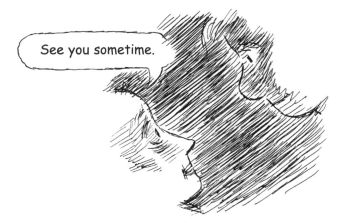

On the twenty-ninth, Janet was awake at intervals, her eyes were yellow with jaundice and had a vague stare, and she was lethargic. That evening, Jane had us switch from the methadone liquid to a pain patch. I was relieved; it was so hard for Janet to swallow.

At night, Janet became agitated. I gave her her 2 a.m. medication early. Then I lay down to sleep behind the couch. Carolyn looked in on her at 4 a.m. Janet continued to be restless in her sleep.

Janet was due to have her pain and anti-anxiety medication at 6 a.m. Usually I got right up. This morning I needed more time. I could hear Auda moving around. I rolled over and called out to her, "I know it's time, I'm just taking another minute more." The next thing I heard was Auda walking over, saying my name:

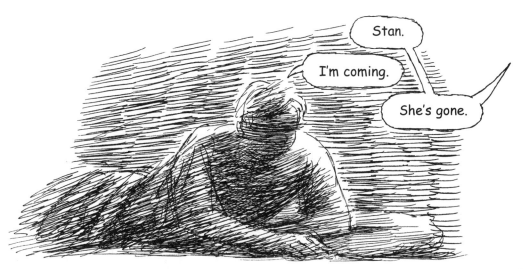

I scrambled up and hurried to Janet's side.

She looked gaunt and silent and her mouth was open. Auda said, "I thought she was sleeping, but I noticed that her belly wasn't moving. I put my hand on her chest and took her pulse. There was none. She went so quietly, she just stopped."

I was trying to put together that I was seeing her dead. That she was dead. All the years and times and life she and I had together rushed over me, all the heartbreaking efforts to hold on to her health and to defeat the illness. Now there was nothing either of us could do.

I pulled up a chair, leaned over the rails, and looked down at her. *Through health and sickness, Janny, till death do us part.*

Carolyn came in and stood next to me and I held on to her and we cried.

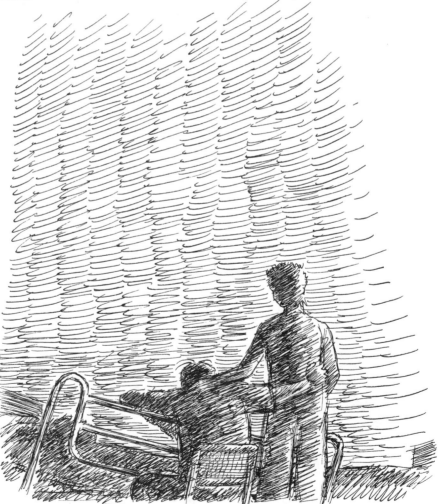

Nichole arrived at 7:30. She and Auda cleaned Janet and dressed her in the purple top, black pants, and purple socks she liked so much. "Gotta be hip." Nichole put on Janet's makeup. I didn't go near the room while they did that.

I knew I had to alert the hospice and funeral parlor. But I was in no hurry. I said to Carolyn, "What's the rush? I want to keep her a little longer."

And I sat with her. Dressed up, she looked peaceful and pretty. But I knew my Janet had packed her bags and hit the road.

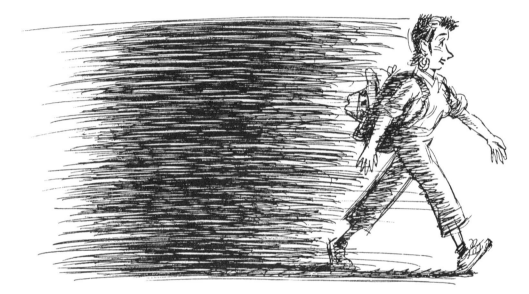

CHAPTER 10

Joke's Over, You Can Come Back Now

That morning the funeral parlor people arrived and gently took Janet's body away. Nichole and Auda stayed and helped. Carolyn handled the phone and the door and draped the hospital bed and commode with a bedspread till we could get rid of them. I have no idea what I was doing.

For a year and a half, for every second of every day, I had expressed my feelings by doing things. Suddenly, there was nothing to do. My hands hung by my sides. The time everyone tried to warn me about was here.

I was alone in a no-man's-land between death and grieving.

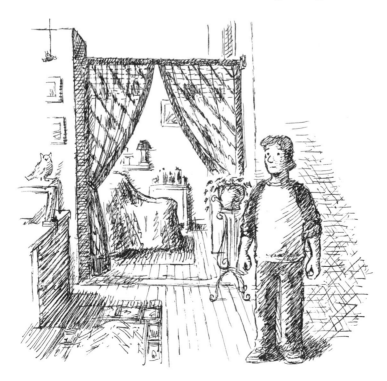

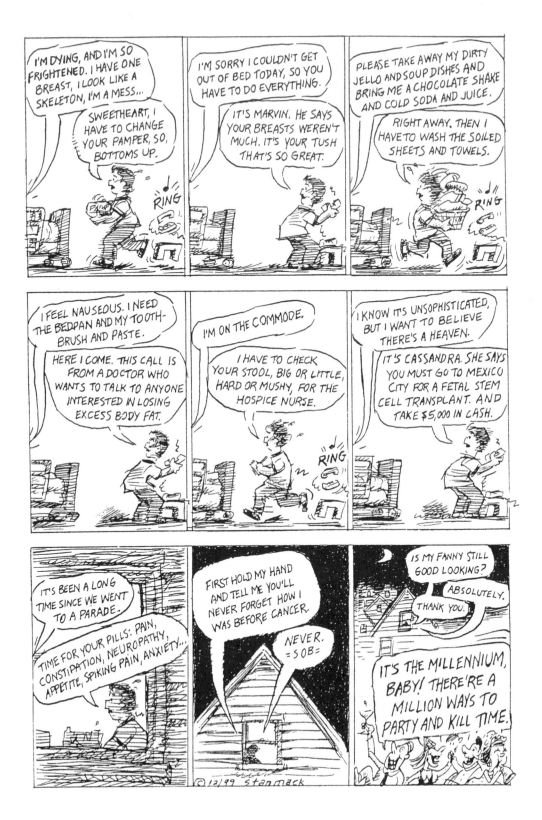

On Sunday, my comic strip appeared in the suburban sections of *The New York Times*. It drew immediate and mostly furious response. Apparently, people sitting down to their Sunday coffee, bagel, and paper did not appreciate being hit with a comic strip about cancer and bowel movements. The editor sent me copies of the e-mails and letters.

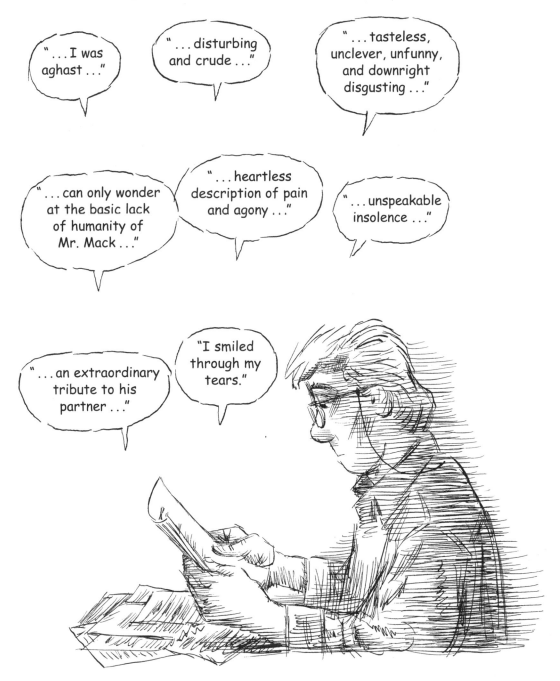

"...I was aghast..."

"...disturbing and crude..."

"...tasteless, unclever, unfunny, and downright disgusting..."

"...can only wonder at the basic lack of humanity of Mr. Mack..."

"...heartless description of pain and agony..."

"...unspeakable insolence..."

"...an extraordinary tribute to his partner..."

"I smiled through my tears."

In the days that followed, the phone kept ringing with calls of support and concern from Carolyn, now back in Los Angeles, and my sister and all Janet's friends. And wonderful condolence notes streamed in through my mailbox.

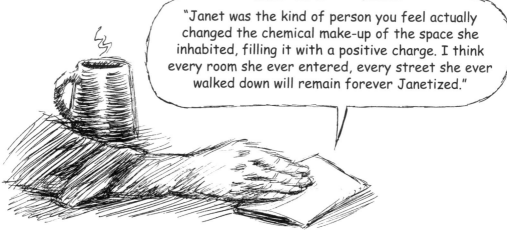

"Janet was the kind of person you feel actually changed the chemical make-up of the space she inhabited, filling it with a positive charge. I think every room she ever entered, every street she ever walked down will remain forever Janetized."

I was numb and probably half insane. Janet's ashes now sat on a shelf in a pretty wooden box. Friends took some of her ashes and in time would take them around the world—to Antarctica, Australia, India, Mali, South Africa, Thailand . . . But I couldn't go near that box. Janet's ghost sat at her computer. Her drawer full of single earrings promised falsely that she'd be right back. I lay awake at 3 a.m., on my egg-crate mattress, eating apples and watching TV.

Physically my body had broken down. I had itchy skin rashes, leg pain, and an erratic heartbeat. And when a doctor told me that I should have a prostate biopsy, I wasn't surprised. I quickly began swearing at the fates for assigning cancer to the same household twice. When the biopsy proved negative, I still figured it was just a reprieve.

I adopted a young cat, thinking that a small beating heart would at least send an arc of warmth into my empty apartment. I named her Picchu. It worked a little, but she was also a pain in the ass, always yelling at me.

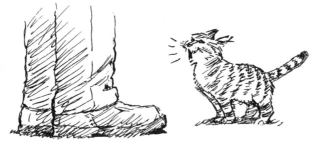

I had two good friends going through divorces. One or the other would drag me to a restaurant or coffee bar where I could be among people who were normal, even if I wasn't.

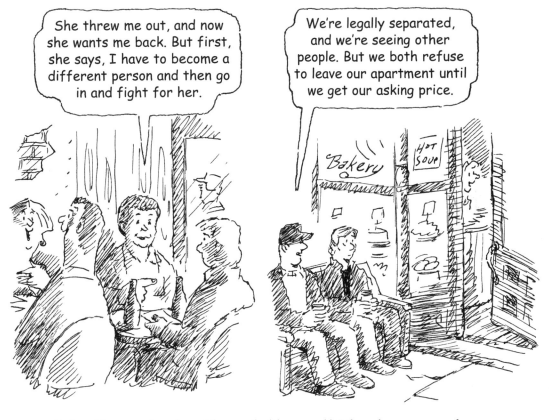

I also felt a need to be with people like myself. I found my way to that hidden world of damaged people who'd been behind those other lighted windows. I'd never been to a shrink or therapy session but, early in January—maybe because it was a short walk away, maybe because I was terribly lonely, and maybe because I wanted to hear other people's stories—I took myself to a bereavement support group.

Gilda's Club provides support, community, and meeting places for people living with cancer. I joined a group who met weekly, mostly women, some men, grieving for parents, spouses, siblings, companions.

Every Tuesday for a year, even when I thought I didn't want to go, I went. We sat in an oval on overstuffed chairs and were led by a facilitator with a light touch and a box of tissues nearby.

We were twenty-five to sixty years old: a manicurist from Queens, a real estate agent from New Jersey, a student from Brooklyn, a TV producer from Greenwich Village, a lawyer from the Upper West Side. Two were left with young children to raise.

There was a Vietnam vet who'd lost his wife and arrived full of an anger that threatened to explode into violence. Instead, the group seemed to calm him and he became a favorite. There was a thirty-year-old woman who'd lost her mother and angrily turned on us for not hurting as much as she. She left after two sessions.

I was secure within this odd circle of people who didn't think they knew better, who let one another talk at length, who could allow extended silence to fill the room, and who gently handed across the box of tissues.

I hadn't known how to take care of Janet. Janet hadn't known how to die. Now I had to learn how to grieve—we all did.

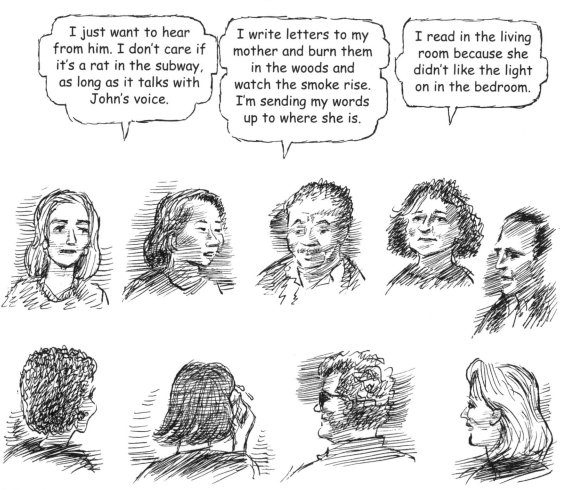

I just want to hear from him. I don't care if it's a rat in the subway, as long as it talks with John's voice.

I write letters to my mother and burn them in the woods and watch the smoke rise. I'm sending my words up to where she is.

I read in the living room because she didn't like the light on in the bedroom.

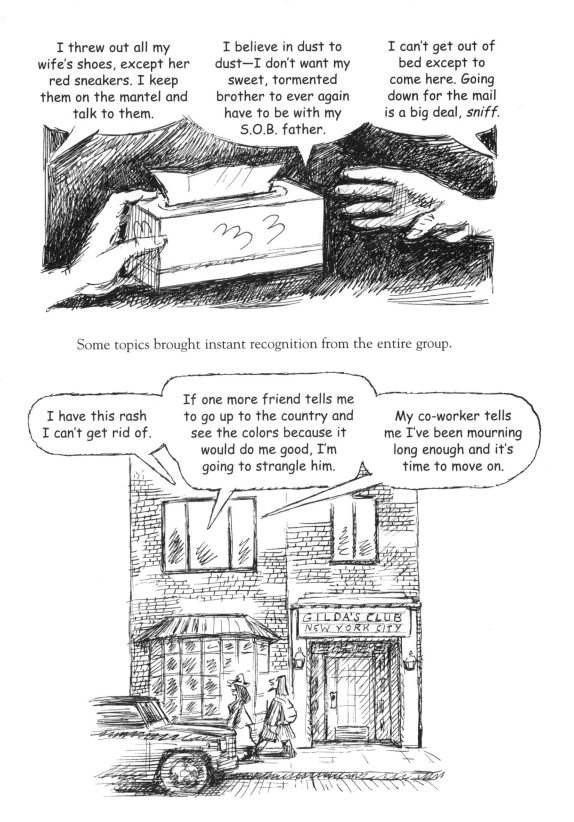

Some topics brought instant recognition from the entire group.

But if we found understanding in that room, during the rest of the week we were vulnerable to ambush from the seemingly insensitive outside world.

While Janet was alive, she and I made all the decisions about her life and illness. We were the inner circle. Everyone else was outside. Now I was on the outside.

I had assumed I would automatically become her executor because she'd named me in her will. But Joe, the estate attorney, hadn't mentioned one detail.

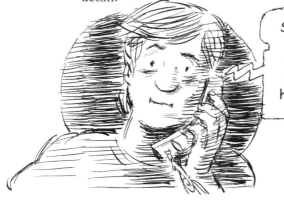

> Stan, you have no authority to marshall her assets until you're appointed executor. I have to first petition the surrogate's court, and the next of kin have to sign a waiver and consent form. But it's just a formality.

Then Lucy's prophetic warning—"Believe me, relatives can get crazy"—came true.

Within a few days, Joe was back on the phone.

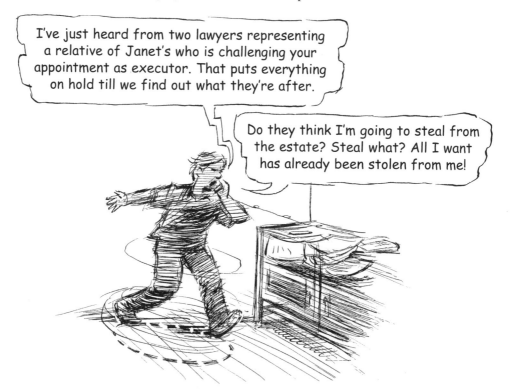

> I've just heard from two lawyers representing a relative of Janet's who is challenging your appointment as executor. That puts everything on hold till we find out what they're after.

> Do they think I'm going to steal from the estate? Steal what? All I want has already been stolen from me!

Now I couldn't get at her money to pay her medical bills or the funeral parlor expenses. I couldn't officially notify her bank or publishers. I couldn't distribute her money to her beneficiaries. The legal challenge was petty, but it held up my appointment for a year.

If we had been married, I would have had some legal standing and many matters would have been easier. Still, Janet and I did what we felt was right for us, and I'm not sorry. Screw 'em!

I still had the joint checking account we'd opened when she was sick. For months I tried to close that account, and every month the bank statement reappeared, with a penalty fee tacked on because I hadn't kept a minimum balance. In the seventh month I snapped.

No problem, sir. You'll get one more statement with a zero balance and that'll be it.

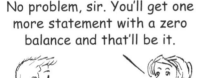

Well, sir, closing an account is not a 1, 2, 3 shot. But you can be confident that the account is now closed.

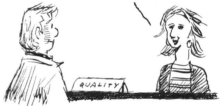

There is one more document the other clerk didn't know about. I'll take care if it.

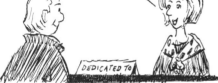

Michael closed it last month? No wonder it was done wrong. But you can depend on me.

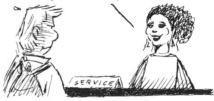

You found it easy enough to open the account! You think you're keeping her alive this way? I'm going to the president of the bank with all your names!

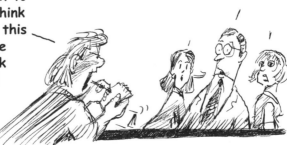

They finally closed it. Janet would have had a field day with them.

Each week I retreated to my group and heard similar tales of woe and was perversely comforted. I sometimes wondered whether God purposely made people stupid in order to distract us from our grief.

"My wife left everything to me. She also loved to dress up and had a walk-in closet full of costume-y clothes. Two weeks after she died, I got a message from her sister saying she was ready to go through the closet. I told her not yet, I wasn't prepared to face it. A month later I was served with a notice that she was challenging the will. Attached was this note:

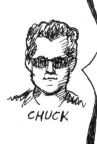

CHUCK

CRASH!

"After all, Chuck, she is my sister. You've only been in her life eleven years. I should get half her clothes and a share of the value of your apartment."

I had coffee with Danny from the group. His wife, Lorraine, died of breast cancer around the same time as Janet. Listening to him was like looking in a mirror.

We would talk in little phrases when she was woozy on medication. I'd whisper, "Who's taking care of you, who loves you?" And she'd always say, "You." A friend said, "Why do you talk gibberish to her?"

I brewed a special herb tea an herbologist had recommended. I even made it in the hospital room. The doctors laughed at what I was doing. One said, "This isn't about nutrition, it's about medical procedures."

The lack of straight talk from doctors came up over and over again in the group. The result was a bitterness toward the medical profession.

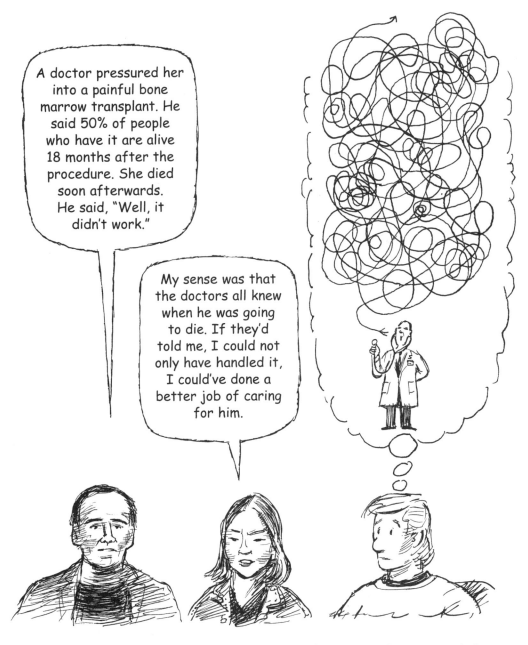

A doctor pressured her into a painful bone marrow transplant. He said 50% of people who have it are alive 18 months after the procedure. She died soon afterwards. He said, "Well, it didn't work."

My sense was that the doctors all knew when he was going to die. If they'd told me, I could not only have handled it, I could've done a better job of caring for him.

These conversations echoed my feelings that Janet's doctors avoided giving us information that would have made what was left of Janet's life easier for all of us.

In researching this book, I talked to the then–executive director of Jacob Perlow Hospice.

"Early in treatment, doctors and patients should have careful conversations about options. Cancer is life shifting, nothing will go back to the way it was before.

"Doctors are there to give it their best shot. But they don't say, 'Where's this patient's head today?' What are they scared of? This is a human being with a life and relationships, so let's bring in referrals. Being supportive is not on their radar. Usually the doctors are hesitant to talk about dying because they feel it will take away hope. But not telling people sets them up for a crisis."

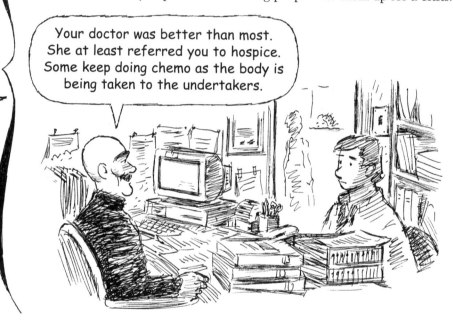

PAUL

Your doctor was better than most. She at least referred you to hospice. Some keep doing chemo as the body is being taken to the undertakers.

I later learned that the hospital Janet went to had a new comprehensive cancer support program in place to go along with standard treatment like chemo and radiation. Now, as soon as the patients enter the hospital, a social worker opens a file on them. They are given information about backup services such as nutritionists, therapists, home health-care aides, and even self-help groups. These services are *prenegotiated* with the patient's insurance company. The philosophy of the program is that the sooner the patients are introduced to the uncertainty of treatment, the better prepared they will be.

The hospital established its cancer support service several months after Janet died.

But finally it was important for me to move past my anger at an insensitive medical profession. Janet had an aggressive cancer and it killed her. Nothing would have changed that. I had to deal with Janet's "gone-ness."

I believed that Janet remained with me in some essential way. It was ridiculous to think that her radiant spirit could just vaporize. She was my guardian angel sitting on an astral perch helping me move on. If it turned out that I had cancer it was because she was going to welcome me to her side sooner. If I were going to go forward in some positive way, it was because she'd had a hand in it.

I remembered her words from the previous November. When Janet was acknowledging the seriousness of her illness, she said to me:

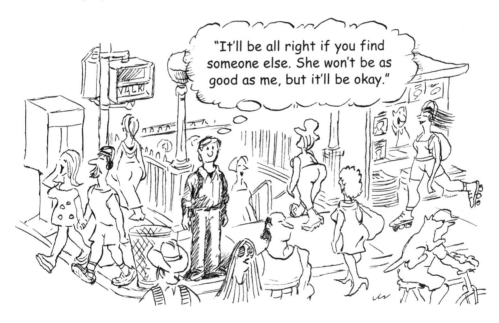

So when the relationship issue came up for me that summer, I was okay with it. However, it was an issue that made the bereavement group uncomfortable.

One evening at our meeting, a man who'd lost his wife reported that he'd just had a date and that they slept together. Most in the room shifted uncomfortably—and this was a bunch who could handle most anything. One woman criticized him, something that was not usually approved of. Another, who'd lost her husband, said she wished she could find a nice man to have a social date with. I kept silent.

In June I'd met a nurse through my hospice friends. We liked each other and over the next two months we went from friendship to a budding relationship. But criticism for who she could never be would creep into my voice. In August, she said, "There's too much of Janet around you." I said, "The last thing I want to do is hurt you."

We agreed to go back to being friends. As we parted, I said, "Your hugs are lethal, you know." And she smiled and said, "Yes."

I had learned something—that I was still alive. I believed that, one day, with the right person, I could keep Janet with me and have another relationship.

I was ready to be positive about my life, but part of me knew that, from then on, Death and I would be drinking buddies.

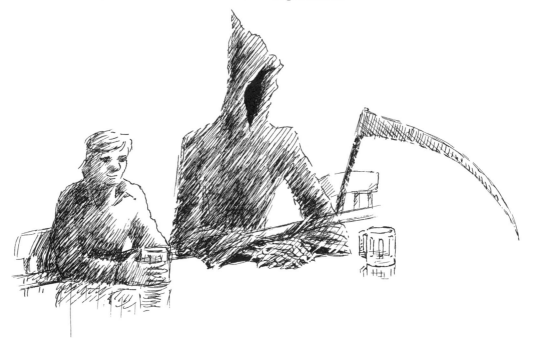

I continued going to the group, but some had left, and there were newer people whose pain was more raw than mine. I was beginning to feel it was time to move on.

By September, I was back in our bed and could again look out at Janet's favorite skyline. I could pick up her earrings and remember the street fairs where we bought them. I could sit at her desk and start the task of going through her files.

Sweet and silly little memories were filtering back in.

Years ago I found a penny on our floor and said, "This is my lucky day."
After that, Janet would leave a coin here or there around the apartment for
me to exclaim over.

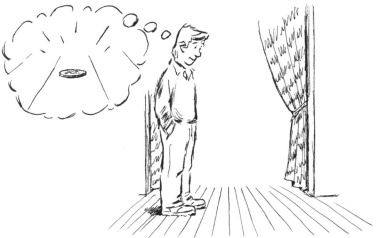

She had opinions on most things, and whenever I was reminded of one,
it made me smile.

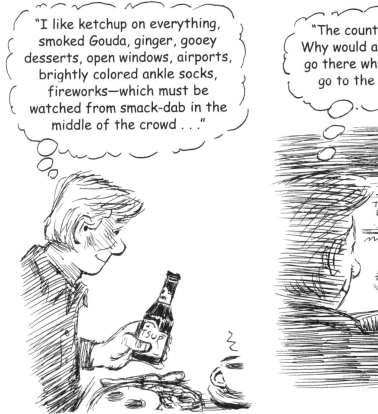

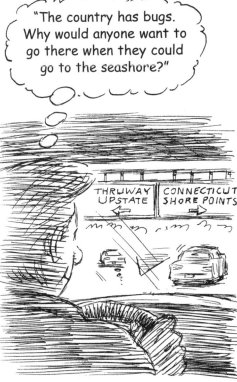

Not that we didn't ever fight, because we did. But after the door slamming and silences, the arguments invariably ended the same way.

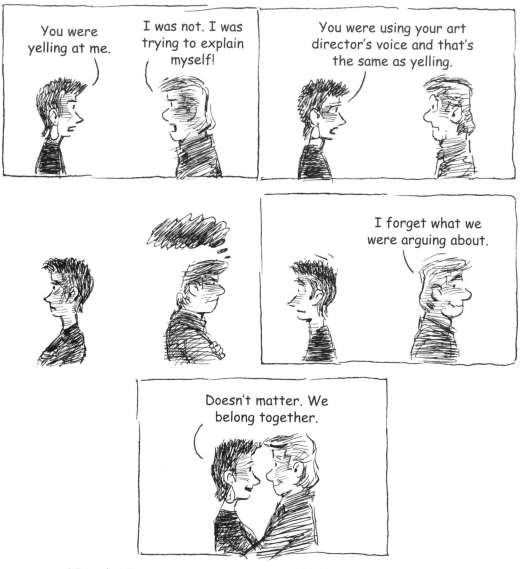

Now that I was stronger, it was time to do what I'd promised myself that I'd do: look squarely at our life together and her illness and death—not duck away, as I'd done when she was sick. I owed it to her and it would help me heal. And, finally, I would write about it—Janet would love that. I'd start by tracking down her friends, sharing stories, crying together.

I made plans to spend some time on the road.

In October I flew to Seattle and met with Jeannie and Bill. I then rented a car and prepared to drive down through Oregon and the San Francisco Bay area and on to Los Angeles. I would track down and spend time with about fifteen of Janet's friends.

She and I had driven that same route twice before. Happy and sad images lay in wait for me everywhere.

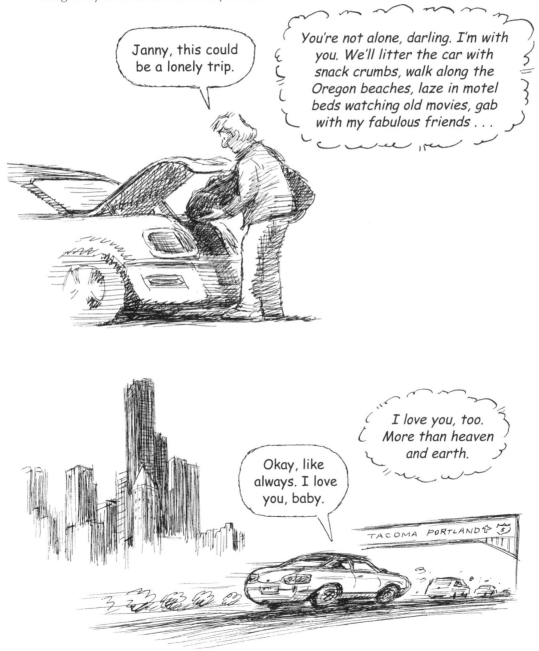

Janny, this could be a lonely trip.

You're not alone, darling. I'm with you. We'll litter the car with snack crumbs, walk along the Oregon beaches, laze in motel beds watching old movies, gab with my fabulous friends . . .

Okay, like always. I love you, baby.

I love you, too. More than heaven and earth.

Forever Janetized

When Janet and I were together, we knew we were meant to be. During the time of her dying, I said I love you every way I could. And all that was not said between us was understood.

Late in the fall, after returning from my West Coast trip, I went biking along the Hudson River. The sky over New York Harbor was that cool blue-gray color that I love.

I watched the slanting rays of silvery light come down through the darkened clouds and thought how life brings both transcendent beauty and terrible pain, without reason.

And that's the way it is. Janet knew that.

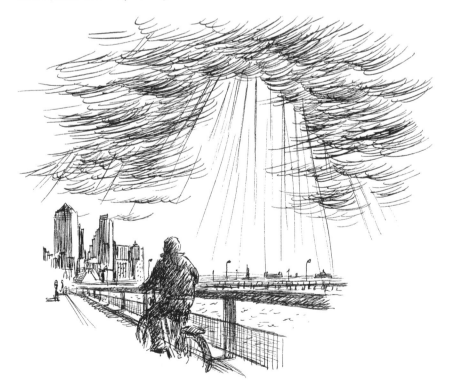

The day after Thanksgiving I woke in the middle of a dream. I was in my apartment. There was a party with people all around. Janet was there but invisible to everyone but me. She was making a salad in the way she enjoyed most, by chopping like mad.

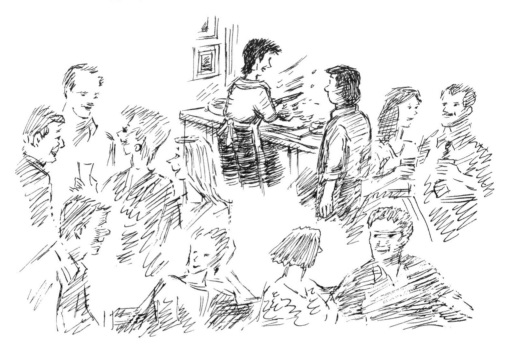

She was animated and normal and seemed okay with the idea that I knew she was really gone. Linda was in the dream and I told her Janet was there. She said:

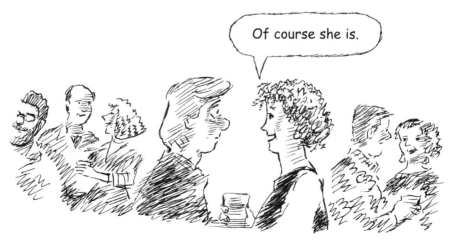

Of course she is.

I remember hugging Janet and being surprised that, even though she was invisible, she was warm and real. It was the first dream of her I'd had in which I could touch her. She smiled and said to me:

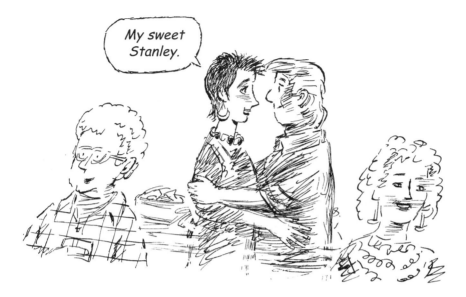

And I thought:

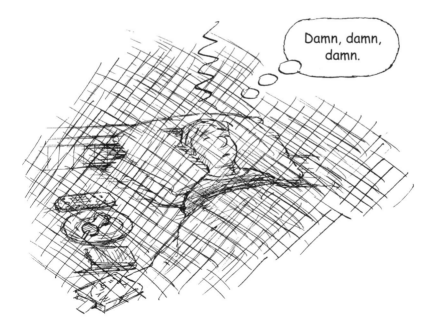

For months after Janet's death, I had lived in the world the two of us created. She was near and I consulted her. As the winter passed, I had the sensation that she was moving further away. Her voice was still there but distant.

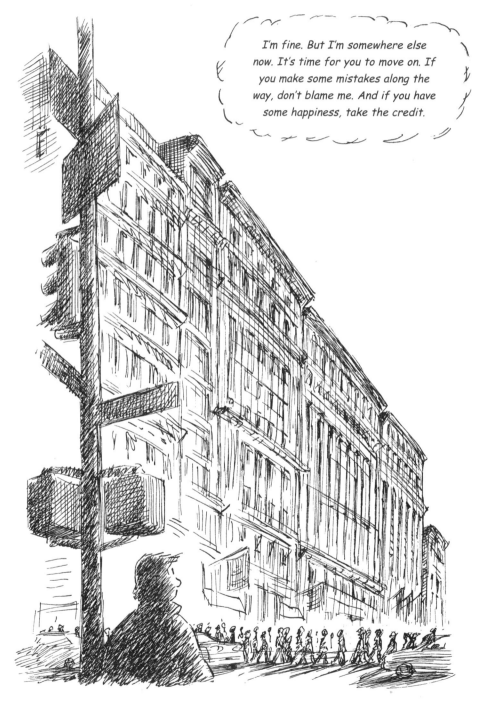

I'm fine. But I'm somewhere else now. It's time for you to move on. If you make some mistakes along the way, don't blame me. And if you have some happiness, take the credit.

Now, when I read a few words that seem an answer to a question I hadn't thought to ask till then, or see fast-moving clouds, or stand on a beach and watch the waves roll in, I know Janet is safe and still with me.

While here on the shore I am a vagabond again.

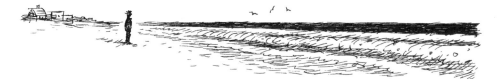

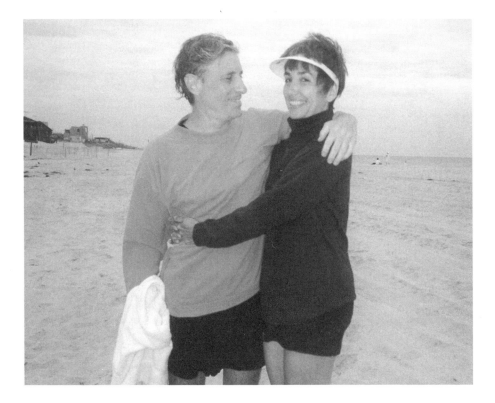

Stan Mack pioneered the form of "real life" cartooning with his notorious New York comic strip *Stan Mack's Real Life Funnies*, which ran in *The Village Voice* for twenty years. He has written and illustrated children's books, teen books with Janet Bode, and two graphic histories, *The Story of the Jews: A 4,000 Year Adventure* and *Stan Mack's Real Life American Revolution*. Mack is the former art director of *The New York Times Magazine*. He is a graduate of the Rhode Island School of Design and divides his time between Los Angeles and New York City.